Weight Management for Type II Diabetes

An Action Plan

Jackie Labat, MS, RD, CDE
Annette Maggi, MS, RD

JOHN WILEY & SONS, INC.

New York • Chichester • Weinheim • Brisbane • Singapore • Toronto

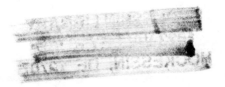

This book is printed on acid-free paper. ☺

Copyright © 1997 by Jackie Labat and Annette Maggi. All rights reserved
Published by John Wiley & Sons, Inc.

Published simultaneously in Canada
Previously published by Chronimed Publishing

The information contained in this book is not intended to serve as a replacement for
professional medical advice. Any use of the information in this book is at the reader's
discretion. The author and the publisher specifically disclaim any and all liability arising
directly or indirectly from the use or application of any information contained in this
book. A health care professional should be consulted regarding your specific situation.

Library of Congress Cataloging-in-Publication Data:

ISBN 0-471-34750-7

Printed in the United States of America

10 9 8 7 6 5

Contents

Introduction

Take action and you can make it happen—that's the motto of this book. No false promises. No guarantees. Just a simple message that puts you in charge of your weight and diabetes management. There are no pat answers when it comes to improving your health. But you can make a difference by taking action.

Weight Management for Type II Diabetes gives you the tools you need to take charge. It walks you through the steps of developing a personalized plan that considers your lifestyle, personality, family situation, and wants and needs. Not only does it factor in lessons for weight management, but it addresses the reason you're trying to lose weight—to improve control of Type II diabetes.

This book helps you assess habits, teaches you techniques of behavior change, and motivates you to find the support you need to manage both Type II diabetes and your weight. It makes sense to tackle both at once. Losing as little as 10 to 20 pounds can improve your control of diabetes.

Additionally, the health habits recommended for diabetes management are very similar to those suggested for weight control—following a low-fat meal plan, becoming more active, managing stress, and developing a support system. By making gradual changes in your habits that you can live with for the rest of your life, you can lose weight and gain better control of your diabetes all at once.

Diabetes control and weight management are a journey—a process continually being worked on—so treat this book as your health journal. Don't just read it cover to cover all in a weekend. Take it slowly and learn about your current habits, changes you need to make, and how to make them. And when you finish the final chapter, keep in mind that you're not really finished. You'll continually be taking action steps to manage your weight and diabetes. After all, as a wise person once said, "Success is a journey, not a destination."

take charge
living with Type II Diabetes

AN ACTION PLAN

You begin by always expecting
good things to happen.
Tom Hopkins

Can you think of times in your life when you looked forward to an event or prepared for something to happen? Take your first day at a new job, for instance, anticipating new faces and different ways of doing things and wondering what the work will be like. "Will I get the hang of it quickly enough?" "What will my coworkers expect?" These are just a few of the questions you might have asked yourself. But once you started, your anticipation subsided, the learning and work began, and the unexpected became the expected—making your new routine a normal part of daily living.

The same anticipation applies to your diabetes and weight management action plan. Whether you were just diagnosed with diabetes or have had it for a long time, you probably have expectations about living with diabetes and the changes in your life you'll have to make. But as you take time to learn the facts, ask questions, and gradually start changing your lifestyle, living with diabetes will seem more doable.

The key is learning what you need to know to help make the unexpected become the expected. In this chapter you'll gain the knowledge you need to understand what Type II diabetes is, who gets it, how you treat it, and the impact of weight loss on overall management of this disease. You'll also learn the steps you can take to create your personal action plan for better health.

Defining Type II Diabetes

Simply put, diabetes mellitus is a chronic disease in which your body can't properly use the food you eat. Normally, when a person who doesn't have diabetes eats, the digestive system changes most of the food into glucose—the body's preferred energy source. Once the food is digested, glucose enters your bloodstream, causing blood glucose levels to rise. Glucose is carried in the blood to cells throughout the body. However, in order for glucose to enter the cells to be used as fuel, insulin needs to be available. Insulin is a hormone made by your pancreas, a gland near your stomach. In response to the rising blood glucose level, the pancreas releases insulin into the bloodstream, causing the glucose to enter the cells and returning blood glucose levels to normal.

Because you have diabetes, however, your body doesn't work as it should. After you eat, your body does break down food into glucose and send it out into your bloodstream, but there are problems with how much insulin your pancreas makes and how well your cells respond to that insulin. The cells in your body don't respond as well to the insulin that's available. They've become insulin resistant. As a result, the glucose can't get into your cells to provide energy, and your blood glucose levels remain high. Eventually, because your body isn't getting the fuel it needs, you start to feel tired and hungry. This process occurs gradually over time. In fact, you may have had diabetes for quite a while without even knowing it.

What causes diabetes? If you're like most people, you may think that eating too much sugar caused your diabetes. Although no one knows the exact cause, it's likely that your genetic blueprint determined whether you would develop Type II diabetes. Your age, extra weight, and inactivity can contribute to the inability of your body to use the insulin it makes, eventually causing you to develop Type II diabetes. People of color—African Americans, Mexican Americans, Asians, Hispanics, and American Indians—are at higher risk for getting diabetes because of genetics, higher rates of obesity, and lifestyle habits.

Can I get diabetes from eating too much sugar?

The exact cause of diabetes is unknown. Diabetes isn't caused by eating sugar. Rather, diabetes is the inability of your body to use sugar (glucose) for energy correctly due to a lack of insulin.

NO QUESTION IS SILLY

Understanding Your Symptoms and Diagnosis

Because the development of diabetes is a gradual process, you may have had diabetes for quite some time before your health care provider diagnosed it. For some people, the initial symptoms are obvious, but for most, they aren't. Diabetes is commonly diagnosed by chance during routine physical exams. At the time of this writing, diabetes is diagnosed when you have one or more of the following symptoms:

> Weakness, fatigue, excessive hunger, extreme thirst, frequent urination, changes in vision, or persistent infections

> Blood glucose levels at 200 milligrams per deciliter (mg./dl.) or higher when checked throughout the day

> Morning blood glucose levels (before you ate) at 140 mg./dl. or higher on at least two separate clinic visits

Knowing the normal blood glucose range for people who don't have diabetes helps put these levels into perspective. When your body produces and uses insulin as it should, your blood glucose levels before eating meals or after fasting should range from 70 to 115 mg./dl. One to 2 hours after a meal, your blood glucose levels should be less than 140 mg./dl.

Managing Type II Diabetes

The overall goal of diabetes management is to keep blood glucose levels within the normal range to prevent or delay long-term complications (for example, heart disease). To do this, the first steps are to change your eating and activity habits. Weight loss, which can result from eating and activity changes, also helps because it improves your blood glucose levels, lowers your blood fats (lipids), and decreases your blood pressure. You'll learn more about monitoring these health parameters in chapter 5.

If your glucose levels don't normalize after you've made lifestyle changes, your health care provider will probably prescribe a glucose-lowering drug. This treatment works best for people with diabetes who still make some insulin, and these medications are designed as a supplement, not a replacement, to lifestyle habits such as being physically active or eating regular meals. Glucose-lowering medications help achieve blood glucose control by increasing the amount of insulin your pancreas produces, improving your cells' sensitivity to the insulin available, decreasing the amount of glucose put out by your liver, or by helping your body to slow down the rate at which it absorbs glucose from food.

If your blood glucose levels remain high after you've made lifestyle changes and started taking a glucose-lowering medication, your health care provider may prescribe insulin injections for you. It could be that your body has stopped making insulin. Like the glucose-lowering pills, insulin can lower blood glucose levels.

How do I know if I have Type I or Type II diabetes?

NO QUESTION IS SILLY

Type I diabetes usually occurs in people under age 20. It affects only 10 percent of all people who are diagnosed with diabetes. Individuals with Type I diabetes produce little or no insulin, whereas those with Type II diabetes still make insulin. Their bodies just don't make enough or use it the way they should. Because people with Type I diabetes don't make insulin, they require daily injections to survive. People with Type II diabetes can often control their blood glucose levels by establishing regular eating habits, becoming physically active, and losing weight. Some, however, may require glucose-lowering pills or insulin injections.

Factoring in Weight Loss

Eating right, increasing activity, and possibly taking a medication for your diabetes are all important steps to achieve blood glucose control, but weight loss helps, too. Losing 10 to 20 pounds improves blood glucose management; your cells become more receptive to the insulin that your pancreas still makes and more responsive to the medications (if any) that you take. This happens because your body uses insulin better, allowing the cells to use the glucose in your blood for energy, which improves blood glucose control. The combination of weight loss and better blood glucose management may even lower the amount of medication you take (if you're currently taking one) or allow you to stop taking the glucose-lowering pills or insulin injections altogether.

A lower body weight may also reduce your risk of weight-related long-term complications associated with Type II diabetes, such as heart disease and high blood pressure. When you lose weight, you can lower blood fats (which put you at risk for developing heart disease) and blood pressure levels. Managing these health parameters helps you prevent or delay other long-term complications of Type II diabetes, such as retinopathy (eye disease) and neuropathy (nerve damage).

Take Control: Climb the Ladder of Health

As you may have anticipated, the goals for managing Type II diabetes are to control blood glucose levels and to manage weight to prevent long-term complications. This book focuses on managing both your diabetes and your weight. It's all one package; the proactive steps you'll take cover both goals. Think of this process as a ladder to climb. Each step up the ladder represents a different component of your diabetes and weight management action plan. What you have to remember is that each rung on the ladder is essential to taking full charge of your diabetes and weight.

diabetes care
stress management
support
monitoring
physical activity
meal planning

The first step on the ladder is meal planning. Your meal plan helps you regulate blood glucose levels, manage weight, and control blood cholesterol levels and blood pressure. In chapter 3 you'll develop a personalized meal plan that fits your lifestyle and allows you to eat a wide variety of foods. Chapter 10 and appendixes B and C give you more detailed information on eating low fat, the different types of fat, and nutrients of special consideration for weight and diabetes management.

The second step on the ladder to good health is physical activity. Activity not only helps you achieve normal blood glucose levels and weight goals but also increases the "good" cholesterol in your body, protecting you against heart disease. Chapter 4 teaches you about the different types of activity with special emphasis on lifestyle activity. It's recommended that you accumulate 30 minutes of physical activity every day. These activities can include walking, taking the stairs, cleaning, and many others. Chapter 9 emphasizes the importance of aerobic, strengthening, and stretching exercises and also teaches you how to stick with your activity plan.

Once you've gotten the basics of food and activity down, you're ready for the next step up the ladder—monitoring. To delay or prevent long-term complications—eye, heart, nerve, and kidney problems—that can develop because of diabetes, you need to monitor blood glucose levels, hemoglobin A1c values (also called glycosylated hemoglobin), weight, blood pressure, and blood fats. In chapter 5 you'll learn more about these terms and what numbers you should try to achieve for improved diabetes management.

Sticking with your program takes daily efforts, and that's why you need support—the next step up your ladder. To be truly successful in maintaining your new lifestyle habits, you need to practice self-care—taking care of yourself—and involve others. Because the changes you're making are likely to impact those around you, it's important to strengthen your program by getting family, friends, and coworkers to support the changes you're making. People who live in supportive environments tend to be more successful at losing weight and maintaining a weight loss. You'll learn more about how to create your support network in chapter 8.

In order to continue managing your diabetes and your weight, you need to learn tactics to cope with stress. Stress management is the next rung on your ladder of good health. Although stress is a normal part of life, stress can make it harder for you to control your diabetes and weight. When you're under too much stress, it's sometimes easy to forgo lifestyle habits you've been working on. Stress can also raise your blood glucose levels. In chapter 14, you'll practice visualization techniques as well as learn the art of positive self-talk. Both will help you cope more effectively with stress and keep the forward momentum going.

What is the difference between glucose and blood sugar?

NO QUESTION IS SILLY

They're actually the same thing. The term *blood sugar* is often used interchangeably with the term *blood glucose*. Glucose is a form of sugar that provides the fuel your body needs to function properly.

Each step you take up the ladder has its own set of beliefs and actions. The most challenging, and yet exciting, step is changing old attitudes and habits to fit your new lifestyle. Behavior change is the support that binds each step of the ladder together. Incorporating each new skill required to manage your diabetes and weight is going to take time, commitment, and daily effort. Although you may spend more time trying to master one of the steps than some of the others, you'll eventually get the hang of it. Chapters 7 and 13 will help you gain the skills you need to maintain your new lifestyle habits and prevent old behaviors from sabotaging your diabetes and weight management goals.

Once you've mastered all the behavior changes required to move up from one rung of the ladder to the next, you'll have achieved the final step—diabetes care. This means you'll be managing your blood glucose levels and weight with the ultimate goal of preventing, or at least delaying, the long-term complications associated with Type II diabetes.

In the chapters ahead, you'll learn all you need to know about managing your weight and diabetes and gain skills that will guarantee success. But first you'll determine if your attitude toward weight management will help or hinder your progress up the ladder of good health and whether you're physically ready to begin leading a more active lifestyle.

I'm worried that my children will develop diabetes. Is there any way to prevent it?

NO QUESTION IS SILLY

Although there is no guaranteed way to prevent diabetes, researchers do believe that making lifestyle changes may prevent your children from getting it. The first step is helping your children manage their weight. If they're overweight, they're four times more likely to get diabetes than a child who is normal weight and has no family members with diabetes. Increasing activity levels is the key. Increased physical activity not only helps children manage their weight but also decreases their blood glucose levels. No studies have found healthful eating to prevent diabetes, but it is important for controlling weight. So whether your children have diabetes or not, your new healthier lifestyle will benefit them.

on your mark, get set, GO

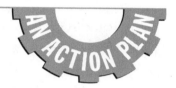

Desire creates the power.
Raymond Holliwell

Living longer, feeling better, preventing the long-term complications of diabetes such as heart disease—these may all motivate you to make changes in your lifestyle. But are you ready to begin your diabetes and weight management program? Do you have the attitude you need to be successful? Will losing weight be any different this time?

The answer to all of these questions can be yes. Yet before you jump in feet first, you'll want to determine your readiness to begin the process of weight management. In this chapter, you'll assess your attitudes about lifestyle habits and weight loss, evaluate your physical readiness to become more active, and examine your weight loss expectations.

Rethinking Your Thinking

Have you ever tried to change a habit—even for a short time—and then returned to old habits? Have you set weight-related goals to please some-one else? Think about it. The only person who can lose the weight is you. If you don't want to do it, you won't.

Before you begin on your weight loss expedition, you need to be absolutely positive you're prepared to make a commitment, a commitment you won't take lightly. Your attitude about losing weight can and will have an impact on your ability to succeed. You need to be realistic with the plan of action you are about to take.

Are You Ready to Lose?

One way to assess your attitude toward weight loss is to take the following readiness questionnaire. For each statement, consider your personal beliefs and indicate whether you believe the answer is true or false.

I've thought a lot about my eating and activity habits and
know what I need to change.　　　　　　　　　　True___ False___

I've accepted the idea that I need to make gradual,
permanent changes in my eating and activity
patterns to be successful.　　　　　　　　　　True___ False___

I'm ready to accept the idea that any weight loss is good
because it can improve my diabetes management.　True___ False___

I know that a gradual weight loss is best.　　　True___ False___

I'm attempting to lose weight for me and no one else
but me.　　　　　　　　　　　　　　　　　True___ False___

I'm ready to commit time and energy to planning and
organizing my meals and becoming more physically
active.　　　　　　　　　　　　　　　　　True___ False___

I know that I can't and won't be perfect in my weight loss
program.　　　　　　　　　　　　　　　　True___ False___

I'm ready to accept that there's no magic answer to
weight loss. I need to come up with a personalized
plan that fits my lifestyle.　　　　　　　　　True___ False___

I have family, friends, or coworkers who will be supportive
of my weight loss efforts.　　　　　　　　　True___ False___

Although answering true to all of the questions doesn't guarantee you're ready to lose weight, the more true answers you have, the more likely you are to experience long-term success. If you answered false to most of the questions, your expectations may not be realistic. Reconsider your weight loss motivations and methods and reassess your readiness to begin a new lifestyle program. Read the upcoming pages carefully and really evaluate what you think about weight management. Learning to focus on the process of losing weight, not the end result (pounds lost), and on self-acceptance is important as you start your journey.

Let's begin by evaluating the "truths" of this quiz. As you reread each statement, consider the meaning of each message. This will help you prepare for the challenge you face ahead.

I've thought a lot about my eating and activity habits and know what I need to change. The more you understand about current behaviors you want to change and the barriers that prevent you from making those changes, the more successful you'll be. In chapters 3 and 4, you'll take a closer look at eating and activity patterns. Chapter 6 will help you set goals to achieve permanent lifestyle changes.

I've accepted the idea that I need to make gradual, permanent changes in my eating and activity patterns to be successful. Some "diets" tell you exactly which foods to eat and when to exercise. Although these may seem helpful initially, they're often too drastic or restrictive compared to your regular lifestyle habits. In other words, they're not changes you can live with on a permanent basis. To be truly successful in diabetes and weight management, you need a program that's customized to your lifestyle, your wants, and your needs, not a program that practices the "one-size-fits-all" philosophy.

I'm ready to accept the idea that any weight loss is good because it can improve my diabetes management. Most people have fantasies of reaching a weight considerably lower than they can realistically maintain. For example, they try to reach their high school graduation weight or fit into a pair of size 8 jeans that are packed away in their closet. Rethink your meaning of "success." A successful, realistic weight loss is one that can be maintained by sensible eating and regular physical activity. A realistic weight also takes

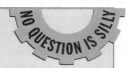

When I start a weight loss program, I often lack motivation to keep going because I lose only 1 or 2 pounds. How do I stay focused?

It's not uncommon to lose motivation when you're trying to lose weight. Weight management is a lifelong endeavor. That's why it's so important to map out small steps toward changing your lifestyle. Take time to think about your past efforts and why they failed. Pinpoint the barriers that kept you from success and create motivational strategies that will keep your momentum going. You also need to remember that it's OK to take breaks from losing weight. Learning to maintain weight is an invaluable tool.

into account your body type. According to the set-point theory, your genetics determine the weight that your body prefers to maintain. Your body will try to maintain this weight no matter what. Family history is also a factor. If your parents are heavier, it's likely you will be.

The goal of weight management is to lose small amounts of weight to improve your health. If you normally weigh 200 pounds, losing 20 pounds can lower blood glucose and blood pressure levels, decrease your cholesterol, and help prevent heart disease.

I know that a gradual weight loss is best. If you've tried diets before, you may be familiar with the term *yo-yo dieting.* Yo-yo dieting is when your weight drops by 20 pounds then 6 months later goes up by 30. A year later, you lose 40 pounds, only to gain it back 2 years after that. Just like a yo-yo, your

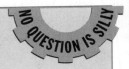

Sometimes I feel as if I have no control over my eating. Several times each week, I find myself bingeing on food. What can I do to make myself stop eating so much?

First it's important to assess your definition of a binge. Webster's dictionary defines a binge as "an unrestrained indulgence." In the medical field, however, the terms *binge* and *binge eating* have specific definitions. The key difference between bingeing and binge eating disorder is whether you feel in control of your eating. If you find yourself eating a large amount of food in a short period of time, you're experiencing a binge. When you eat too much too fast, feel as if you can't stop eating (even if you wanted too), and feel depressed or guilty after eating, you may have what's called binge eating disorder.

If you feel out of control when you binge, talk about these issues with your health care provider. Your provider can refer you to a mental-health professional and a registered dietitian for help. Binge eating disorder is treatable. Treatment includes three steps. First, change your disordered eating patterns. This involves eating three meals a day with snacks and learning to listen to your internal hunger and satiety (fullness) cues. Second, identify and change how you feel about your weight and body shape and about food itself. Third, learn how to identify triggers in your environment that make you feel like bingeing and learn to manage these situations. The goal of therapy for binge eating disorder is decreasing the number of times you binge. In the long run, you'll be more successful with weight management if you take time to get help and learn to manage the binge behavior.

weight goes up and down—typically by 20 pounds or more from year to year. Instead of trying a short-term, quick-fix diet, it's best to lose weight gradually by not cutting calories down too fast and by combining activity and lifestyle habits with healthful eating for permanent weight loss.

Emphasis on gradual weight loss is essential. Aim for 1/2 pound to 1 pound per week as the maximum goal and remember that as long as you're maintaining your weight (not gaining weight), you're still making progress. Ideally, try to focus on the process of losing weight (the development of positive new lifestyle habits). Take one day at a time and make daily choices to achieve your results.

I'm attempting to lose weight for me and no one else but me. It's often easier to tell yourself you're losing weight for your spouse, doctor, or perpetual dieting friend. But does losing weight for someone else really work? Think back and you'll probably agree that only you have the answers on the best way for you to lose weight. You need to come up with a plan that works for you. You're the one who has to live with the new lifestyle you're about to create and make the day-to-day decisions—not someone else.

I'm ready to commit time and energy to planning and organizing my meals and activity schedule. Weight loss doesn't just happen. It takes time and energy. You'll need to start by assessing your current lifestyle, evaluating potential barriers that may prevent you from achieving your goals, and planning for success. Realize that the program you are about to embark on may not be easy—yet long-term diabetes and weight management are well worth the effort.

I know that I can't and won't be perfect in my weight loss program. Do you know anyone who eats perfectly and always sticks with his or her activity program? Expecting perfection is like planning for failure. Too often people get caught in the all-or-nothing mentality when they decide to lose weight. It's important that you learn to be gentle and forgiving of yourself. You can anticipate that there will be lapses—times when you slip back to old lifestyle habits. It's all a matter of how you react to setbacks. Learn from them and move on. You have to keep that forward momentum going.

I'm ready to accept that there is no magic answer to weight loss. I need to come up with a personalized plan that fits my lifestyle. There is no quick fix to weight management. Putting on weight takes time, and losing weight definitely takes time. You may have heard of the "Grapefruit Diet," the

"Cabbage Soup" diet, or supplements such as chromium picolinate touted as increasing your metabolism. No pill or special food can make you lose weight easier or faster—these diets and supplements can also be detrimental. You need to design a realistic program that fits your lifestyle and personal needs.

I have family, friends, or coworkers who will be supportive of my weight loss efforts. Having support doesn't guarantee you'll lose weight, but it does improve your chances for success. Asking for support from others can help you get what you need and keep you on track. Whether sharing the weekly task of grocery shopping, exercising with a friend, or talking during stressful times, each situation brings you one step closer to your long-term weight and diabetes management goals.

Are You Physically Ready?

Now that you've assessed your attitudes about losing weight, it's time to evaluate your physical readiness. Physical activity is a key component in your weight and diabetes management plan. Complications of diabetes, medications you're taking, and your current lifestyle habits can all affect how you go about managing your weight and diabetes. For example, most people think it's OK to start exercising suddenly after years of being sedentary. However, if you have nerve or eye damage, there are additional health risks to consider. To decide if you should pay your health care provider a visit before you start making changes in your activity level (chapters 4 and 9), complete the following quiz.

Evaluate Your Health Risks

Are you over age 40 and sedentary?   Yes___ No___

Have you had Type II diabetes for 10 or more years?   Yes___ No___

Do you have uncontrolled high blood pressure?   Yes___ No___

Has your health care provider ever told you that
    you have heart trouble?   Yes___ No___

Has anyone in your immediate family had heart disease
    or a stroke before age 60?   Yes___ No___

Do you ever feel pain in your chest?   Yes___ No___

Has your health care provider ever told you that you have
    a bone or joint problem such as arthritis that could be
    aggravated by exercise?   Yes___ No___

Do you ever experience shakiness, dizziness, sweating,
    faintness, blurry vision, or headaches?   Yes___ No___

Have you had high blood glucose levels over the past
    several months?   Yes___ No___

Do you experience low blood glucose levels regularly?   Yes___ No___

Do you experience shortness of breath or breathlessness
    after daily activities?   Yes___ No___

Has your health care provider ever told you
    that you have nerve damage?   Yes___ No___

Do you have eye disease related to your diabetes?   Yes___ No___

If you answered yes to any of these questions, you should call your health care provider to see if you need a complete physical exam before you begin changing your activity level. Do this as soon as possible so that you're truly ready to embark on your new lifestyle program. Being active means you'll feel better, improve your health by controlling blood glucose levels, and be more successful in losing and maintaining a weight loss. You'll learn more about the benefits of activity and how to change your activity level in the upcoming chapters.

Set Reasonable Weight Goals

The third and final evaluation of your readiness to begin your weight management program is determining whether your weight loss goals are realistic. For example, if the lowest weight you've reached as an adult is 170, it's unlikely you'll be able to drop to 150 pounds. Here are some tips to help you be realistic with your weight loss goals:

Consider your family history. If one or both of your parents are overweight, it's likely that you'll also weigh more than height and weight charts suggest.

Review your personal weight history. What was your lowest adult weight? What was your highest adult weight? Ideally, you'll want to set a weight goal that you can achieve and maintain without starving yourself or exercising excessively. It should be a weight that you maintained in the past for at least one year without struggling. If you've always been overweight, think about the lowest weight you've ever been able to achieve and whether maintaining that weight is realistic for you now.

Start small. Remember, a 10- to 20-pound weight loss can improve your diabetes management. Today's recommendations encourage you to lose 10 percent of your weight. So multiply your weight by 0.10 to get an initial goal. For example, if you weigh 200 pounds, your initial weight loss goal

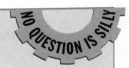

I've heard that there are now pills I can take to lose weight. Wouldn't this be the easiest and quickest way to help my diabetes control?

Appetite suppressant drugs, such as dexfenfluramine (Redux) and phentermine and fenfluramine (phen/fen), may help you lose about 5 to 15 percent of your current body weight. These drugs work by increasing your brain levels of serotonin—a chemical that is thought to control how full you feel. When your appetite is suppressed, you eat less.

What you may not know is that once you start taking the medications, it's likely you'll take them for the rest of your life. That's because once you go off these medications, weight gain slowly resumes, especially if you don't work on lifestyle changes. Whether you take medications or not, the basics of weight management—low-fat eating, leading an active lifestyle, and behavior change—still apply.

As simple and wonderful as these drugs sound, as with any other medication, there are side effects associated with taking them. Because these drugs affect the levels of serotonin in the body, they can make depression worse. They can also cause sleep disturbances, dry mouth, diarrhea, and nervousness. People who take these drugs are also at higher risk for pulmonary hypertension. This rare, life-threatening condition results in increased pressure from the artery to the lungs. The effects of taking these obesity medications for more than a few years aren't known.

If you're interested in these medications, talk with your physician to see if they're appropriate for you.

would be as follows: 200 pounds × 0.10 = 20 pounds. If you feel the need to break it down further, aim for losing 1/2 pound to 1 pound per week. Once you achieve the 20-pound weight loss, practice maintaining the weight for several months before trying to lose weight again. Keep in mind that you want to focus on making positive lifestyle behavior changes, not on weight. In chapter 15 you'll learn how to be successful at maintaining your weight loss.

Use height and weight charts as your last resort. If you or your health care provider is really determined to set goals based on height and weight charts, keep them in perspective. These charts only give guidelines. They can't take into account your personal weight history or your genetic blueprint. If you can't achieve a weight in the goal ranges, you can still be healthy and improve your diabetes control.

In coming chapters you'll learn how to develop the habits necessary to lose weight, improve your diabetes management, and enhance your overall quality of life. Although you may associate losing weight with deprivation and loss, keep in mind that it doesn't have to be this way. Times are changing, and so are you. This isn't another diet plan—a diet has a beginning and an end. The program you're trying to achieve consists of gradually making healthful lifestyle changes, and assessing your readiness was the first step.

Earlier in the chapter, you were encouraged to focus on the process of losing weight, not the outcome (weight loss). Change is a process. Initially, making lifestyle changes is difficult because internally there is often resistance to changing old habits. Bear in mind that by reading this book and actively participating, you are planning for change. Each succeeding chapter will arm you with knowledge, self-assessment tools to build new and improved habits, and motivation to continue on your weight loss journey. By taking one step at a time, you're more likely to accomplish your goals and reap the health rewards of success.

designing your own meal plan

He who has a *why* can bear almost any *how*.
Friedrich Nietzsche

AN ACTION PLAN

Eat less. Weigh less. These statements have been ingrained in your brain by the media. Pick up any magazine at a grocery store counter and you'll find headlines such as "Lose 10 Pounds in 10 Days" or "Slim Your Waistline." If you've tried any of these quick, restrictive, weight loss diets, you've probably been unsuccessful at achieving permanent weight loss. You may even be reluctant to try another program. After all, most diets didn't work and left you feeling deprived. Yet this time, you have some additional motivation: you want to lose weight and eat better to manage your diabetes.

Reality is that managing your weight and diabetes requires more than just eating less food or avoiding sugar. It's about the type and amounts of food you eat, consistency in mealtimes, and a host of other factors. It's also very individual. What works for one person may not work for you. That's the focus of this chapter—10 simple steps to designing a meal plan that meets your needs, fits your lifestyle, and helps you achieve diabetes and weight management.

Step One: Keep a Food Journal

Changing your eating habits is possible only when you know what habits need modifying. Because it's hard to remember exactly what you eat each day, a journal or written record is the best way to accurately identify eating patterns that prevent you from achieving your health goals. When you take the time to write down when and what you eat, you get accurate feedback that can be used to modify lifestyle habits.

In order to notice patterns in your eating habits, keep detailed records for at least three days. Use the next 3 pages to record what and how much you eat. Try to record two weekdays and one weekend day. Your eating schedule is also important when you have diabetes, so make sure you record the time when you eat your meals and snacks. The information you'll get from these records will help you develop strategies tailored to your individual needs, lifestyle, and time demands.

Most people tend to change their food choices and the amounts they eat when they have to write them down. This is a natural tendency; everyone wants his or her eating habits to look great when they're printed in black and white. This exercise will be most effective, however, if you're honest with yourself and eat normally during the days you're recording. Carry the record with you and fill it out during meals. Remember to record snacks and "extras" such as butter, gravy, dressing, and sauces added during cooking or at the table.

Once you've completed your 3-day food record, begin looking up the calories and fat grams of the food you ate. Refer to appendix A for additional fat and calorie counts. You can also use the Nutrition Facts food label found on most products. (You'll learn more about this in chapter 11.) After you've recorded the fat and calories for each food item, total your daily fat grams and calories. You'll use this information later in the chapter.

The Daily Food Record—Example

After each meal and snack, fill in the time, food eaten, and amount. Later, add calorie and fat gram information from appendix A, food labels, or other published lists.

TIME	FOOD EATEN	AMOUNT	CALORIES	FAT GRAMS
12 p.m.	whole wheat bread	2 slices	160	2
12 p.m.	sliced chicken	1 oz.	47	1
12 p.m.	mayonnaise	1 tbsp.	100	11
Daily Totals:				

The Daily Food Record

After each meal and snack, fill in the time, food eaten, and amount. Later, add calorie and fat gram information from appendix A, food labels, or other published lists.

TIME	FOOD EATEN	AMOUNT	CALORIES	FAT GRAMS

Daily Totals:

To record additional days, photocopy this page.

The Daily Food Record

After each meal and snack, fill in the time, food eaten, and amount. Later, add calorie and fat gram information from appendix A, food labels, or other published lists.

TIME	FOOD EATEN	AMOUNT	CALORIES	FAT GRAMS

Daily Totals:

To record additional days, photocopy this page.

The Daily Food Record

After each meal and snack, fill in the time, food eaten, and amount. Later, add calorie and fat gram information from appendix A, food labels, or other published lists.

TIME	FOOD EATEN	AMOUNT	CALORIES	FAT GRAMS

Daily Totals:

To record additional days, photocopy this page.

Step Two: Analyze Your Food Records

Next, assess your eating habits using the Eat Smart Quiz. Review your food records and look for patterns in when, how much, and what types of food you're eating. Check one answer from row 1, 2, or 3 for each food choice and total the number of checks for each row. Refer back to your food record as needed to take the quiz.

Eat Smart Quiz

Meals and Snacks

- ❏ 1. I skip meals each day.
- ❏ 2. I eat 2 meals and some snacks each day.
- ❏ 3. I eat 3 meals and snacks each day.

Meal Timing

- ❏ 1. I eat meals at different times each day.
- ❏ 2. I occasionally eat meals at about the same time each day.
- ❏ 3. I usually eat meals at about the same time each day.

Bread, Cereal, Rice, and Pasta Group

- ❏ 1. I eat 2–3 servings each day.
- ❏ 2. I eat 4–5 servings each day.
- ❏ 3. I eat 6 or more servings each day.

Vegetable Group

- ❏ 1. I don't eat vegetables.
- ❏ 2. I eat 1–2 servings each day.
- ❏ 3. I eat 3 or more servings each day.

Fruit Group

- ❏ 1. I eat 1 serving each day.
- ❏ 2. I eat 2 servings each day.
- ❏ 3. I eat 3 or more servings each day.

Meat, Poultry, Fish, Dry Beans, Eggs, and Nuts Group

- ❏ 1. I eat 5 or more servings each day.
- ❏ 2. I eat 3–4 servings each day.
- ❏ 3. I eat 1–2 servings each day.

Milk, Yogurt, and Cheese Group
❏ 1. I eat no dairy products.
❏ 2. I eat 1 serving each day.
❏ 3. I eat 2–3 servings each day.

Fats and Oils
❏ 1. I eat 8 or more teaspoons of margarine, butter, oil, mayonnaise, and regular salad dressings.
❏ 2. I eat 5–7 teaspoons of margarine, butter, oil, mayonnaise, and regular salad dressings.
❏ 3. I eat 4 or fewer teaspoons of margarine, butter, oil, mayonnaise, and regular salad dressings.

Sugary Foods (table sugar, honey, candies, soft drinks)
❏ 1. I eat sugary foods daily.
❏ 2. I eat sugary foods every other day.
❏ 3. I eat sugary foods only occasionally.

Desserts (cookies, cakes, pies)
❏ 1. I eat desserts daily.
❏ 2. I eat desserts every other day.
❏ 3. I eat desserts only occasionally.

Check the foods you typically eat:
❏ 1. whole milk
❏ 2. 2% milk
❏ 3. skim milk

❏ 1. high-fat cheeses like Colby, jack, cream cheese, Swiss, cheddar
❏ 2. medium-fat cheeses like mozzarella, feta, farmers, string cheese
❏ 3. fat-free cheese

❏ 1. ribs, corned beef, hot dogs, sausage, bacon, salami, peanut butter
❏ 2. ground beef, beef or pork roast, pork chops, lamb, tuna packed in oil
❏ 3. lean pork or beef, chicken, turkey, tuna packed in water, shrimp, ham, Canadian bacon

❏ 1. chips, nuts, and butter- or cheese-flavored crackers
❏ 2. low-fat snack foods
❏ 3. fat-free snack foods

Step Three: Rate Your Eating Habits

Now that you've completed the evaluation of your eating habits, you can assess how they stack up. If most of the checks in the Eat Smart Quiz are next to number 3s, you're doing a great job; your eating habits are in line with a healthy lifestyle. Checks by the number 2s indicate you've made a good start at eating healthfully. If most of your checks are next to number 1s, changes in your eating habits are essential for your health and well-being. Even small changes you make will help you lose weight and improve your diabetes management. As you read on, refer back to your answers on the quiz to determine what changes you're willing to make so that eventually more and more of your checks are beside the last answers.

Step Four: Establish Consistent Eating Patterns

Refer back to the daily food record you kept for three days to see if there are any patterns in when you eat. You might also review your answers to the first two questions on the Eat Smart Quiz—meal timing and skipping meals. If you've always eaten three meals and snacks each day, maintain this routine. Eat breakfast, lunch, and your evening meal at about the same time each day. This helps keep blood glucose levels from going too high or low and regulates your appetite so that you're less likely to overeat. If review of your food records suggests you are a constant snacker or eat six small meals, you may need to make some changes in your meal timing. Consistency is the key. Try to schedule snacks at least 2 to 3 hours before a meal. Spaced meals and snacks improve your body's ability to use insulin, allowing your blood glucose levels to rise and fall before you eat again.

Step Five: Determine Your Fat and Calorie Budget

Once you've assessed your current eating patterns, it's time to learn how to design your own weight loss plan for improved diabetes control. Many people have lost weight by simply trimming the amount of fat they eat because fat has twice as many calories as do carbohydrates and proteins. So by limiting fat, you can eat just as much food yet get fewer calories, and this helps you lose weight. A low-fat diet can also keep your blood lipids in check. You'll learn more about them in chapter 10. Keep in mind, however, that a low-fat meal plan shouldn't be considered a free-for-all. Too many calories, whether from carbohydrate, protein, or fat, will lead to weight gain.

To calculate your typical fat and calorie intake, refer back to your 3-day food record for additional information. Using the following chart, determine your average daily calorie and fat gram intake as well as the percent of calories you're getting from fat.

Calculating My Fat Budget

	CALORIES	FAT GRAMS
Day 1		
Day 2		
Day 3		
Total		
divided by 3 (to get average) =		

$$\frac{\text{average fat grams} \times 9}{\text{average calories}} = \% \text{ of calories from fat}$$

$$\frac{\times 9}{\underline{\hspace{3cm}}} = \underline{\hspace{1.5cm}} \% \text{ of calories from fat}$$

If your percentage of calories from fat is between 20 and 30, you're already in your goal fat gram range and on your way to losing weight. If more than 30 percent of your calories are coming from fat, don't be discouraged. Simple, gradual changes in the food choices you make can be very effective at lowering the amount of fat you eat.

So where do you start? What does "eating low fat" actually mean? You can begin by counting fat grams in everything you eat until you get a feel for the amount of fat in various foods. Continue to refer to appendix A and food labels. You can also refer to appendixes B and C for more information. Appendix B, "The Enlightened Shopping Tour," will help you make low-fat choices at the supermarket. Appendix C, "The Low-Fat Cooking Lesson," provides ideas on how to lower the fat in some of your favorite recipes.

In addition to counting fat grams, don't forget to count calories. Although today's fat-free and low-fat world makes it easier to keep your fat budget down, fat free doesn't mean calorie free. If you want to be really successful at achieving weight loss and diabetes management, you need a program that consists of both fat and calorie counting.

To find an appropriate calorie level for you, start by subtracting 250 calories from the average daily calories you calculated from your food records. This will promote about a 1/2-pound-per-week weight loss. Once you're comfortable at this reduced calorie level, you may want to subtract an additional 100 to 250 calories from your average daily calories on page 27. However, keep in mind that to get all the nutrients the body needs, women should drop no lower than 1,200 calories a day and men no lower than 1,500 calories.

When establishing a calorie level, remember that this is a pattern you want to be able to follow for the rest of your life. New lifestyle habits are your goal, not a 3-month "diet." So focus on a plan that allows you to eat less gradually but still feel satisfied.

The amount of fat you can have each day depends on the number of calories you eat. Major health organizations recommend that no more than 30 percent of calories come from fat. The goal, however, is not zero fat. To lose weight, keep your fat intake at 20 to 30 percent of daily calories. If your current fat intake is above 30 percent, set your initial goal at 30 percent. Once you're comfortable at this level, you can eliminate more sources of fat from your food choices (see appendixes B and C for ideas). If you're already at 30 percent, make 25 percent your goal. Again, assess where you're currently at and what simple, gradual changes you can make in your eating habits. Don't deprive yourself by trying to go too low, too fast. Taking small steps is truly the way to succeed in long-term weight and diabetes management.

These percentages are useful when looking at your overall eating habits, but what you need for day-to-day practicality is your fat gram budget. The following table lists daily calorie goals and the total fat grams that represent 20 to 30 percent of the total calories. Find the calorie level in the first column that is closest to what you have estimated as your goal calorie intake. Then, in the other columns, find the amount of fat recommended for your calorie level. This is your daily fat gram budget.

Step Six: Eat a Wide Variety of Foods

Counting fat grams and calories, although essential for weight loss, doesn't guarantee you'll eat nutritious foods. To achieve the perfect balance of nutrients, you need to eat according to the Food Guide Pyramid (see the

Daily Fat Gram Goal

CALORIE GOAL	30%	25%	20%
1,200	40	33	27
1,300	43	36	29
1,400	47	39	31
1,500	50	42	33
1,600	53	44	36
1,700	57	47	38
1,800	60	50	40
1,900	63	53	42
2,000	67	56	44
2,100	70	58	47
2,200	73	61	49
2,300	77	64	51
2,400	80	67	53
2,500	83	69	56

My daily budget is _____ calories and _____ fat grams.

next page)—a pyramid of five food groups and a "use sparingly" group.

Bread, Cereals, Rice, and Pasta Group: Enjoy 6 to 11 servings a day, depending on the total number of calories that is appropriate for you. One serving equals 1 slice of bread, 1/2 cup cooked rice, pasta, or cereal, or 1 ounce ready-to-eat cereal.

Fruit Group: Eat 2 to 4 servings each day. One serving equals 1/2 cup raw (chopped), cooked, or canned fruit, 3/4 cup fruit juice, or 1 medium apple, banana, or orange.

Vegetable Group: Aim for 3 to 5 servings each day. One serving equals 1 cup raw leafy vegetables, 1/2 cup cooked or raw vegetables, or 3/4 cup vegetable juice.

Meat, Poultry, Fish, Dry Beans, Eggs, and Nuts Group: Choose 2 to 3 servings each day. One serving equals 2 to 3 ounces of cooked lean meat, poultry, or fish. Count the following as 1 ounce of meat: 1/2 cup cooked dry beans, 1 egg, or 2 tablespoons peanut butter.

Milk, Yogurt, and Cheese Group: Eat 2 to 3 servings each day. One serving equals 1 cup of milk or yogurt, 1 1/2 ounces of natural cheese, or 2 ounces of process cheese.

Fats, Oils, and Sweets Group: Eat sparingly. There's no "requirement" for these calorie-rich foods, many of which have little or no nutritional value.

To keep fat and calorie intakes down, choose low-fat and fat-free foods from each category of the pyramid. Remember that each of these five food groups provides some of the nutrients your body needs. No one food group is more important than the other. For good health, you need them all. If you have received a meal plan from your health care provider or dietitian, follow the plan specifically developed for you, noting that the portion sizes may be different than those listed in the Food Guide Pyramid.

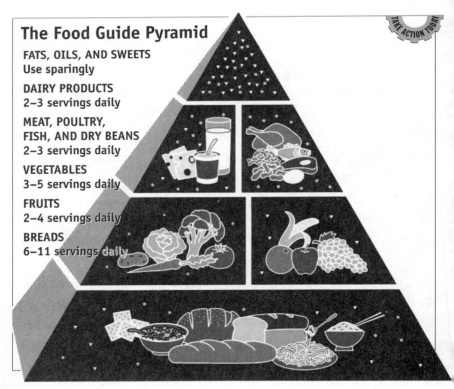

The Food Guide Pyramid

TAKE ACTION TODAY

FATS, OILS, AND SWEETS
Use sparingly

DAIRY PRODUCTS
2–3 servings daily

**MEAT, POULTRY,
FISH, AND DRY BEANS**
2–3 servings daily

VEGETABLES
3–5 servings daily

FRUITS
2–4 servings daily

BREADS
6–11 servings daily

Step Seven: Eat a Proper Mix of Carbohydrates, Protein, and Fat

When you eat according to the Food Guide Pyramid, you get the appropriate balance of the major nutrients—carbohydrates, protein, and fat—that your body needs. Ten to 20 percent of your daily calories should come from protein, and the remainder of your calories should come from carbohydrates and fat. You'll want to eat a much higher proportion of carbohydrates than fats because your goal is to lose weight.

Carbohydrates. Carbohydrates are the energy source your body prefers. They are found in the milk, vegetable, fruit, and grain groups in the Food Guide Pyramid. If you've had diabetes for a while, you might have been taught that there are simple and complex carbohydrates and that these have different effects on your blood glucose. Current recommendations if you have diabetes, however, emphasize that whether you eat a slice of bread or a cookie, both will affect your blood glucose. The key difference is that the nutritional value of a slice of bread is far superior to that of a cookie. Complex carbohydrates such as breads and grains are also high in fiber. Fiber-rich foods make you feel full without overloading on calories and may help lower your blood cholesterol level. You'll read more about the benefits of fiber in chapter 10.

Because all carbohydrates affect your blood glucose level, you'll want to try to balance your carbohydrate choices throughout the day. In addition to monitoring food portions, you should monitor the number of carbohydrate servings you eat at each meal. Meal plans that spread out foods such as milk, fruits, and breads give the best blood glucose response. So try to eat a consistent number of servings from the fruit, milk, and bread groups

I eat consistent amounts of carbohydrates at meals, but sometimes I still find that my blood glucose levels vary quite a bit after eating. Why?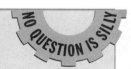

Other factors can affect how fast different carbohydrates raise your blood glucose levels. For example, portion sizes, the amount of fat or protein you ate at your meal, the amount of medication in your body (if you take one), your activity level before eating, and what your blood glucose level was before you ate all can cause your blood glucose levels to be higher or lower than normal.

of the Food Guide Pyramid at meals and snacks. For example, aim for 3 to 4 choices from these groups per meal and 1 to 2 servings per snack. Remember to count sweets, too. If you have a cookie or some ice cream, substitute these for other carbohydrate-containing foods at your meal rather than eating them in addition to your meal. Doing this will help you maintain consistent blood glucose levels.

Protein. The meat and dairy groups of the Food Guide Pyramid are the main sources of protein in your meal plan. Although protein can be used by your body indirectly as an energy source, the rest is used for other functions of the body such as building and repairing muscle. People who have diabetes don't need any more protein than people who don't have diabetes. In fact, most people eat too much protein, which makes their kidneys work extra hard to get rid of waste. As a person with diabetes, you want to avoid eating extra protein because you're more at risk for developing kidney problems. To delay kidney problems, try replacing animal proteins with vegetable proteins (vegetables, grains, beans).

You also don't want to eat large quantities of meats or whole-milk dairy products because they not only are high in fat but also contain saturated fat, a type of fat that increases your blood cholesterol level, contributing to your risk of developing heart disease.

Fat. Fat is one nutrient you've probably heard a lot about in recent years. Fat—especially animal fats or hydrogenated fats—can contribute to heart disease, which is much more common in persons with diabetes. Although you do need to eat some fat, most people eat too much. Remember, fat has

---

If I buy fat-free foods, do I need to limit my portion sizes?

NO QUESTION IS SILLY

It's a common misperception that fat free means calorie free. If you eat more calories than your body needs, you will gain weight regardless of whether the calories come from fat or carbohydrate. Many of the fat-free foods are also higher in carbohydrates, which will affect your blood glucose control. Fat free also doesn't guarantee that a food is nutritious. The grocery store aisles are loaded with fat-free brownies, cookies, muffins, and other desserts. Although these foods are great for occasional treats, they should not replace foods such as fruit that contain fiber, vitamins, and minerals.

twice as many calories as do carbohydrates or protein (9 calories per gram versus 4 calories per gram for carbohydrates and protein). So less fat means fewer calories. Chapter 10 will discuss the different types of fat in greater detail.

Step Eight: Practice Portion Control

Many persons with diabetes are surprised to learn that one of the most important aspects in regulating blood glucose levels and controlling their weight is eating moderate portions of different foods. As mentioned earlier, it's important to eat about the same amount of carbohydrates (fruits, breads, and milk) at meals and snacks to regulate blood glucose levels. At the same time, it's surprising how an extra ounce of meat or pat of margarine can add up to an extra few hundred calories over a week's time. This is just enough calories to prevent weight loss and throw off that good blood glucose control you've been working toward.

To learn portion sizes, measure foods every day for at least 1 to 2 weeks. Use measuring cups and spoons. If you have a scale, you can weigh meats—typically 3 ounces is the size of a deck of cards. You can also read portion sizes on food labels (see chapter 11 for more information). Once you feel comfortable knowing the size of your bowls, plates, and glasses, you can reduce the frequency of measuring and weighing to once a week or on an "as needed" basis.

Step Nine: Keep Tracking What You Eat

The key to healthful living, diabetes management, and weight loss is balance, moderation, and consistency. In order to change and achieve new, permanent eating habits, it's important to continue monitoring what and when you eat. So keep tracking!

Make additional copies of the Fat and Calorie Control Work Sheet (page 36)—one for each day. List the foods eaten, calories, and grams of fat. Using the work sheet, assess whether you're eating a variety of foods from the food groups. For example, if you eat an apple, note that you ate one serving from the fruit group of the Food Guide Pyramid. At the end of each day, add up calories and fat grams and check your balance among the food groups. Remember that your weekdays and weekends may be different. To get a true picture, you need to look at both.

You'll also want to keep in mind that it's common for the amount of fat you eat to vary from day to day. Your goal is to keep the average amount of fat you eat over a 1-week period within your fat gram budget. This gives you flexibility, too. If you know you have a business luncheon or a party where higher-fat food choices will be served the following day, you can cut back on fat grams the day before in an effort to balance your total daily fat grams.

If the thought of daily tracking seems overwhelming, start by doing it every other day and work your way up to daily tracking. Once you become more familiar with the fat and calorie content of different foods, you'll find you don't need to record on a daily basis. Return to recording if you reach a plateau, experience a weight gain, or feel yourself slipping back into old eating patterns.

How much sugar am I allowed each day?

You don't need to avoid sugar totally. Sugary foods should, however, be substituted for other foods that contain carbohydrates (such as breads and fruit) when eaten at meals or snacks. Don't eat sugary foods in addition to your normal food choices. You'll also want to keep in mind that many high-sugar foods are also high in fat and have little nutritional value.

I frequently buy sugar-free candy as treats. Because it is sugar free, can I eat as much of it as I want?

No food should be eaten in unlimited quantities. Sugar-free candies can be incorporated into your meal plan in moderation. Many sugar-free candies are made from sugar alcohols such as sorbitol, mannitol, and xylitol, which can cause diarrhea if eaten in large amounts. You also need to keep in mind that some sugar-free foods are still high in carbohydrates—it's just a different form of sugar.

Step Ten: Putting It All Together

You've taken time to review your current eating habits and examined how to lose weight and improve your blood glucose levels. Next, take a few moments to prioritize what you've learned and decide what changes in your eating habits need to happen. Current nutrition recommendations for people with diabetes emphasize eating consistent amounts of carbohydrates at meals and snacks at similar times each day. So if you're not doing this already, you have your first step. Once you've started regulating blood glucose levels, then you can focus on eating less fat, fewer calories, and a variety of foods.

As you continue to record what you eat, take time on a regular basis to revisit the following questions. These questions are designed to help prioritize the important steps you need to take to improve your blood glucose and weight management. So start slowly and work through each question to achieve positive lifestyle habits.

What times of day do I usually eat? Do I frequently skip meals?

How is my total day's food intake distributed throughout the day? Am I spreading my carbohydrate choices (fruit, milk, and bread groups) evenly between meals and snacks?

Do my portion sizes need to be adjusted?

Am I staying within my fat gram budget? If not, should I add fat grams for a more realistic goal now and lower it once I am comfortable at this slightly higher level?

What foods from my food records were high fat? Are there low-fat substitutions I can make that will still be satisfying to me?

Do I eat a variety of foods throughout the day, or am I missing any of the food groups?

Once you've identified areas you would like to change, you can start developing new habits. Chapter 6 will teach you how to set appropriate goals. The secret is learning to identify the changes you'd like to make and then begin to eat more consciously. Gradual changes in your eating patterns will contribute to your long-term success.

Fat and Calorie Control Work Sheet

TAKE ACTION TODAY

FOOD EATEN	AMOUNT	CALORIES	FAT GRAMS	FOOD GROUP

Daily Totals:

To record additional days, photocopy this page.

activate your health

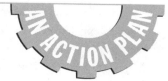

AN ACTION PLAN

The greatest of all mistakes is to do nothing because you can only do a little. Do what you can.
Anonymous

There's definitely more to managing your diabetes and weight than just watching what you eat. Study after study shows that physical activity is the missing link. People who get moving and keep moving are more successful at losing weight and maintaining their weight loss. In fact, regular physical activity seems to be the strongest predictor of success.

Why is activity important for weight management? Because your body weight—to some degree—is regulated by the number of calories you eat and the number of calories you use each day. In order to maintain your weight, you need to burn the same number of calories you eat. To lose weight, you need to burn up more calories than you eat. When you lead an active lifestyle, you burn up excess calories that would otherwise be stored as fat.

So how much activity is enough to manage weight and improve diabetes control? Contrary to what many people believe, you really don't need to do that much. For example, if you weigh about 180 pounds, you could burn 150 calories grocery shopping, 180 calories weeding flower beds, or 220 calories stacking wood—all in 30 minutes. Add that up over a week's time, and you could burn 1,000 to 1,500 calories just from 30 minutes of daily lifestyle activity.

Yet most people don't get moving because they think they have to do high-intensity activities such as aerobics classes or running. They don't realize that even small amounts of activity done consistently add up to big health gains. The key is getting started. In this chapter, you'll discover the benefits of being active, learn the difference between exercise and physical activity, gain a better understanding of the five types of activity necessary for an all-star program, and begin to design your own personal activity action plan.

Reap the Health Rewards of an Active Lifestyle

Physical activity, which is any bodily movement that requires energy, is the first step toward an active lifestyle. Believe it or not, accumulating 30 minutes of lifestyle activities such as taking the stairs, going for a brisk walk, raking leaves, or cleaning the house on most, or all, days of the week is another important step toward managing your weight and diabetes. Being active helps you improve your overall health, lose weight, lower your blood glucose levels, prevent heart disease, and refresh your outlook on life.

At this point, you might be saying, "I don't get it. What's the difference between physical activity and exercise?" Exercise is a more vigorous type of activity that involves planned, structured, and repetitive body movements that are done to improve your body composition (body fatness), flexibility, muscular strength, as well as your heart and lungs. Jogging, step aerobics, swimming, and biking are just a few examples of exercise. All activity—whether it's in-line skating, lifting weights, stretching, or daily lifestyle movements such as taking the stairs or washing dishes—improves your health. Just look at all the benefits you can get from being active:

Activity improves diabetes management by

decreasing the need for diabetes medications,

helping your body use diabetes medications better, and

reducing your blood glucose levels.

Activity helps you maintain or lose weight by

reducing body fat,

controlling your appetite,

increasing your metabolism, and

burning calories.

Activity can lower your risk for developing serious health problems by

> increasing your "good" cholesterol (HDL),
>
> lowering your blood pressure,
>
> preventing osteoporosis (brittle bones), and
>
> protecting against colon and breast cancer.

Activity can enhance your quality of life by

> improving your sleep pattern,
>
> reducing stress,
>
> increasing your energy levels,
>
> boosting your self-esteem, and
>
> helping you feel better about your body.

Can simple physical activity really help me? I've always been told "no pain, no gain."

NO QUESTION IS SILLY

Despite what health club ads on TV say, you don't need to sweat and strain yourself in order to get health benefits from activity. All activities burn calories, improve your sleep, and provide the many health benefits listed in this chapter. In fact, if you experience pain, something is wrong.

Developing an All-Star Activity Plan

Knowing the benefits of leading an active life can be motivating, but it doesn't automatically change your activity habits and daily routine. You need to take action steps to attain success—and the first step can be the hardest. One of the biggest mistakes is to do nothing because you feel you can't do enough. Remember, doing something is better than doing nothing. Your activity goal is to do whatever you can.

Sometimes changes need to be so small you don't even notice them. On a clear night have you ever looked up at the sky and noticed the stars mov-

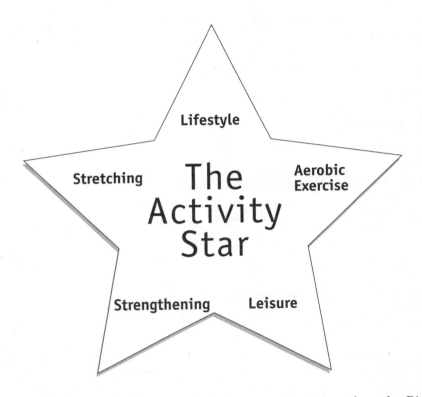

Lifestyle

Stretching

The Activity Star

Aerobic Exercise

Strengthening

Leisure

ing through space? When you look for constellations such as the Big Dipper, have you ever noticed that their location and shape are slightly different from season to season? Although you may not be aware of the Earth's and star's constant motion, these changes do happen. And they happen slowly. Think of your activity plan in the same manner. You want to make gradual changes that feel comfortable—not overwhelming—and add up to big changes over time.

Continue to visualize a star. Every star has five points, and so does your activity program. These include lifestyle, leisure, aerobic, stretching, and strengthening activities. No star is complete without all five points, and neither is your activity program. You need them all.

Lifestyle activities are the first point of your all-star program. If you've been sedentary, work to increase your day-to-day activities. Try getting off the bus a few blocks early and walking the rest of the way to work. Be active at home: sweep and scrub the floors, mow the lawn, vacuum the rugs, or trim the shrubs. Everything counts!

Once you've started moving, add fun leisure activities such as golf, hiking, tennis, dancing, canoeing, or kayaking. Start by incorporating one each week to add variety, feel energized, and stay motivated. As you become more active, work up to a few each week.

The next all-star activity is aerobic exercise. It not only conditions your heart, lungs, and muscles but lowers your blood glucose levels and burns calories. Aerobic activities involve rhythmic motion of your arms and legs. Biking, jogging, walking, cross-country skiing, in-line skating, and swimming are good examples. Your ultimate goal—as you slowly add to your routine—is to exercise aerobically three to five times per week for 20 to 60 minutes.

Before and after aerobic exercise, don't forget to stretch. Stretching exercises help you perform daily motions more easily by improving your muscle flexibility and joint mobility (which reduces your risk of injury). Although most people include stretching exercises as part of their aerobic workout, it's recommended that you do stretching exercises every day— even on days when you don't work out.

Strengthening exercises—which include lifting weights, doing push-ups and sit-ups, and using resistance or rubber bands—are the final point of your all-star program. Everyone needs muscular strength, whether you carry a book bag, briefcase, 40-pound bag of dog food, or small child. Strength conditioning helps make these day-to-day activities easier to perform by decreasing bone and muscle loss as well as reversing weakness that commonly occurs with aging—enhancing activity levels as you get older. Try to include these movements on an every-other-day basis.

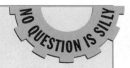

I'm still a bit confused. Does my aerobic exercise count as part of the recommended 30 minutes of physical activity each day?

Physical activity is any bodily movement that requires energy, and exercise is a structured form of physical activity. So the answer is yes, aerobic exercise can be counted toward your goal of getting 30 minutes of activity each day. You want to become more active on a day-to-day basis, whether it's lifestyle or aerobic exercise. However, to maximize the amount of weight you lose and receive the greatest benefits for your heart and diabetes, you'll want to get daily lifestyle activity and aerobic activity three to five times per week.

All-Star Activity Log

ACTIVITY	MINUTES	TOTAL
walk to and from car	10	
(4 times)		
ballroom dancing	20	
shopping at the mall	20	50 min.

Monday

Tuesday

Wednesday

Thursday

Friday

Saturday

Sunday

How Do You Rate?

To determine how active you are and whether you need to make some changes, track your activity level for the next seven days using the All-Star Activity Log on the previous page. Record the types of activities you currently do each day and the number of minutes. Total your minutes of activity for each day in the third column of your log.

Once you've recorded your activity for seven days, review your All-Star Activity Log and answer the questions on the following Rate Your Activity Level Quiz.

Rate Your Activity Level Quiz

To complete this quiz, refer back to your All-Star Activity Log. Assign points for each category as indicated. Total your score to see how you're doing.

Lifestyle   _____

Give yourself a point for each day you did 30 minutes of lifestyle activities.

Leisure   _____

Give yourself a point for each day you did any leisure activity.

Aerobic   _____

Give yourself a point for each day you did 20 to 60 minutes of aerobic activity.

Stretching   _____

Give yourself a point for each day you stretched before exercising or after a workout or participated in activities such as yoga or tai chi.

Strengthening   _____

Give yourself a point for each day you lifted weights, did push-ups or sit-ups, or used an exercise band.

Add up your score. **Total** _____

Now evaluate your score. If your score is:

Less than 7: Work to increase your present activity level by adding lifestyle and leisure activities first. Start gradually and focus on being consistent. Review the five points of your all-star activity program and the tips on page 49, Twenty Ways to Increase Activity, for ideas on how to lead a more active lifestyle.

7 to 15: You've started the foundation for your five-point activity plan. Make sure you're incorporating a wide variety of activities each week. All types of physical activity—whether it's lifestyle or aerobic exercise—are essential for improved health, weight management, and well-being.

16 or more: Congratulations! You've achieved an all-star activity program. Work to maintain it!

A Word to the Wise

Before you jump on the activity bandwagon, there are a few steps to take before you start becoming more active. If you're over age 40 and have been living a sedentary lifestyle, or if you have any complications of diabetes, such as heart disease, high blood pressure, neuropathy, or retinopathy, check with your health care provider to determine if you have any exercise restrictions. Refer to the assessment tool you completed in chapter 2 to see if you have any preexisting conditions that would prevent you from exercising.

Make sure you have some type of identification on you at all times that indicates you have diabetes. To get an ID bracelet, check with your local chapter of the American Diabetes Association (the phone number will be in your local telephone book) or ask at a jewelry store, pharmacy, or medical clinic.

If you take insulin or an oral medication for your diabetes, it's best to do aerobic exercise when your blood glucose levels are the highest, such as one or two hours after a meal, to avoid hypoglycemia (low blood glucose levels). You may even want to check your blood glucose before you begin. If it's lower than 100 mg./dl., have some fruit or a bagel as a snack. Carrying some carbohydrates with you also helps in case you start to feel dizzy or faint—the symptoms of low blood glucose levels. A few options are juice, crackers, or glucose tablets.

Getting Started: It's as Easy as 1-2-3

No matter where you're at with activity and exercise, it's important to have a plan of action on how you'll start, gradually increase, or maintain your current routine. The key is developing a program that incorporates all five points of your star: lifestyle, leisure, aerobic, stretching, and strengthening exercises. More importantly, they should be activities that you enjoy so that you'll continue doing them!

Look back over the quiz and the types of activity described in the previous section. Are there some leisure activities listed that you enjoy but aren't doing? Do you need to increase your lifestyle activity or add a few more minutes to your brisk walk to meet the recommended amount of aerobic exercise?

Take a moment now to list up to three things you can do to lead a more active lifestyle over the next two weeks:

1. _____

2. _____

3. _____

Now, think about your schedule for the next two weeks. At a minimum, plan to maintain your present activity level. Then consider if you can realistically add any—or all three—of the activities you have listed into your schedule. If you've been very active, continue to plan a variety of activities every week. Whatever level you're at, grab your calendar now so that you can make appointments with yourself to be active. Record your plan for the next two weeks on the log provided or on the calendar you use for all your other appointments.

Example Week

Sunday—cleaning 30 minutes

Tuesday—water aerobics 1 hour

Thursday—walk on treadmill 30 minutes

Saturday—Stretch while watching TV

Week 1

Sunday

Monday

Tuesday

Wednesday

Thursday

Friday

Saturday

Week 2

Sunday

Monday

Tuesday

Wednesday

Thursday

Friday

Saturday

If you're having trouble thinking of new ideas or are unsure of how to increase your present activity level, here are 10 Take Action Today strategies to help you build more activity into your lifestyle.

Take Action Today

Make it playful. Children get physical activity instinctively by playing. Think back to your childhood. What activities did you enjoy? Did you like sports and active recreation? You can join an athletic league such as tennis, bowling, golf, volleyball, flag football, or softball. Try bike riding, jumping rope, or basketball, too.

Participate in seasonal activities. Each new season brings a host of activities along with it. During the summer, try in-line skating, hiking, canoeing, or horseback riding. In the winter, if you live where there's snow, enjoy snowshoeing, ice-skating, or skiing. During poor weather conditions, opt for indoor walking at a shopping mall, line dancing, squash, karate, or an aerobics class. Varying your choices will keep your routine interesting.

Choose activities you enjoy. Most people think that being active can't be fun. If you don't try a variety of activities and find some you like, you won't stick with it.

Be realistic. It doesn't matter if you get your lifestyle activity by accumulating 30 minutes throughout the day or in one 30-minute session. Do whatever fits into your routine. Consistency is the key.

Make it a priority. Include ideas for increasing lifestyle activity into your daily "To Do" list. You may even want to schedule activity on your calendar so that you rank it as a top priority along with other work.

Find ways to become more active. You can pace or do some stretching exercises while talking on the cordless telephone, do leg lifts when sitting at your desk, squeeze a stress ball when stuck in traffic, or do sit-ups when watching TV. All of these activities can add up to 30 minutes when done over a day's time. Review Twenty Ways to Increase Activity on the next page for ideas.

Keep an activity log. Record your activities each day to assess whether you're meeting your goals. If you are, congratulate and reward yourself. If not, develop a plan that helps you get more activity.

Remind yourself of the many benefits of leading an active lifestyle. Activity improves your diabetes management, helps you control your weight, prevents chronic diseases such as heart disease, and makes you feel better about yourself. Generate reasons to get activity every day.

Find a partner. Enjoy being active with a family member or friend. Explore a park, walk around a lake, or play a leisurely game of golf. It's easier to be accountable to someone else.

Do I need to buy special shoes before becoming active?

NO QUESTION IS SILLY

For any type of exercise, it's essential that you wear the proper shoes and socks. If you have problems with calluses on your feet, or if you're flat-footed, for example, you may need custom-made inserts that only a podiatrist (foot specialist) can prescribe. Additionally, as a person with diabetes, you're more likely to have nerve problems in your feet (neuropathy) or poor circulation (peripheral vascular disease).

When buying shoes, shop later in the day and start by trying on shoes designed for each sport (for example, walking or running shoes). You need different types of support depending on the types of activities you do. Make sure you have plenty of room for your toes—about 1/2 inch between your longest toe and the end of the shoe. Shoes should be snug, not tight. Try to get a pair with a soft insole and inner lining. Avoid shoes that have thick seams. Wear athletic socks that have padded heels and toes for protection. They should be made of a material, such as acrylic, that takes perspiration away from your skin. And don't forget to walk around the store with the shoes on and check for comfort. If they aren't comfortable in the store, it's likely they won't be comfortable when you get them home.

Pace yourself. If you've been very inactive, start out slow. Maybe your goal should be 10 minutes of activity per day or 30 minutes of activity a few times a week. Build up to 30 minutes all, or most, days of the week. The key is to start with where you're at today and make improvements.

Maintain the Momentum

To make your activity plan successful over time, continue to evaluate where you're at and where you want to go. In chapter 6 you'll learn how to set realistic, manageable goals. Remember that making activity a part of your daily routine takes time. It's just like brushing your teeth; once you get in the habit, it's easy to stick with it. Doing it consistently is what really counts.

Twenty Ways to Increase Activity

Walk around the block every time you get the mail.

Pace or stretch when talking on a cordless telephone.

Play with your children or dog.

Explore a local park.

Plant a vegetable or flower garden.

Take dancing lessons.

Walk before or after work, or at lunch.

Treat your dog to two short walks every day.

Visit a local arboretum or zoo.

Be a little less efficient with housework—make extra trips when picking up.

Take the stairs instead of the elevator.

Hide the remote and walk to the TV to change channels.

Play racquetball or basketball.

Do leg lifts or sit-ups while watching TV.

Park at the far end of the parking lot.

Get off the bus a block or two before your destination and walk.

Go ice-skating or cross-country skiing.

Clean the attic, basement, or closets.

Trim your trees and shrubs.

Stretch every morning when you get out of bed.

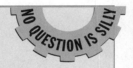

I have small children at home, and caring for them often makes getting aerobic activity difficult. Any suggestions?

If you have very young children, you can walk them in a stroller or buy an attachment for your bicycle so that they can pedal with you. You can try exercising to aerobic videos, using a stationary bicycle, or, depending on your budget, walking on a treadmill. Check with your local health club, as many offer child care while you work out. Try alternating with your neighbors—take turns baby-sitting with them—so that you can be active.

monitoring counts

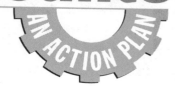

Take time to look, then time to change.
Jane Stephenson

By designing a personalized meal plan and starting to get active, you're on your way to improved diabetes management and long-term weight control. But before you move too far along on your journey, consider the importance of monitoring. Tracking and recording certain aspects of your health provides you with a glimpse of how well you're doing with your overall care plan. Monitoring also tells you when it's time to take actions toward change. For example, if your blood glucose levels are too high or too low, your health care provider may need to adjust your medications. Or perhaps you're eating too much or too little. Without records of blood glucose levels and notes on day-to-day changes in your eating or activity routine, it's difficult to pinpoint the exact cause.

So monitoring is to your advantage. It helps you maintain tight control of your diabetes and weight to prevent or delay the complications of diabetes. In this chapter, you'll learn about these health complications and gain an understanding of what you need to monitor to prevent or delay them. Blood glucose levels, the hemoglobin A1c test, changes in body weight, blood lipids, and blood pressure are the health parameters recommended for you to monitor. Each of these tests reflects how well you're doing with the lifestyle changes you're making.

Understanding Long-Term Complications

If you're like most people, one of the toughest parts about diabetes is understanding all the terms associated with the disease—especially the long-term complications. You might not be clear about how they develop or understand what having them means. Over the years, if your blood glucose levels are uncontrolled, you can develop retinopathy (eye disease), heart and blood vessel disease (heart attack, stroke), nephropathy (kidney disease), and neuropathy (nerve disease). Skin, feet, and dental problems are also common complications of diabetes. Listed here are some definitions to help you improve your understanding of what the terms mean.

Retinopathy. Although most people with diabetes may never develop serious eye problems, a common concern for people who have had diabetes for 25 years or more is retinopathy—a disease of the retina. Diabetes weakens tiny vessels that supply the retina (the light-sensing tissue at the back of the eye) with blood. Eventually the blood vessels may swell and leak fluid, hindering your retina's ability to accept images and resulting in blurred vision or even sudden loss of vision.

Nephropathy. About 10 percent of people with diabetes develop kidney problems (nephropathy). Kidneys filter waste products out of your blood and excrete them in your urine. If your blood glucose levels consistently run high over the years, the small blood vessels in your kidneys can become damaged and lose their ability to filter blood effectively. When they can't filter your blood, harmful waste products build up, causing kidney disease.

Heart Disease. As a person with diabetes, you're twice as likely to develop cardiovascular (heart) disease. You're at even greater risk if you have high blood pressure, use tobacco, have high total cholesterol levels, low high-density lipoprotein (HDL) levels, are overweight, or lead a sedentary lifestyle.

Neuropathy. Throughout your body, a network of nerves carries electrical messages to different body parts, telling them what and how you feel. If you scald yourself with water, get a sliver, or step on a rock, the nerves in your body tell your brain, and you react. If your blood glucose levels are not well controlled over the years, your nerves can become damaged. When nerves are damaged the messages may not get sent or received correctly; they get mixed up. For example, you may not feel a cut on your foot, or you could feel pain in a part of your body even though there isn't anything wrong.

Health Checks

Although the thought of developing these complications may seem overwhelming, the good news is that when you manage blood glucose levels and lose weight, you lower your chances of getting these conditions. To achieve these goals, it's important to monitor the following five health parameters: blood glucose levels, hemoglobin A1c, weight, blood lipids, and blood pressure.

1. Managing Blood Glucose Levels

To prevent or delay long-term complications, you need to maintain blood glucose levels within your goal range. In chapter 1, you learned that people who don't have diabetes have fasting blood glucose levels in the range of 70 to 115 mg./dl. Because you have diabetes, your goal range will be a little different. In the morning, your fasting blood glucose should be less than 150 mg./dl. During the day (1 to 2 hours after meals), your blood glucose should remain less than 180 mg./dl. Your health care provider can give you further guidance on what "normal" is for you.

In order to keep blood glucose levels under control, it's important to know when changes in blood glucose take place, how to treat them, and, most important, how to prevent them from happening. Because your

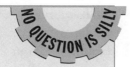

I'm changing my eating habits and losing weight, but now I'm experiencing more low blood glucose levels. What causes this?

Losing weight, getting more active, and changing your eating habits can all cause your blood glucose levels to become somewhat irregular. One reason for this may be that the level of medication you take (if you use insulin or glucose-lowering medications) is no longer appropriate. If you are experiencing low blood glucose levels (hypoglycemia) more often, or find yourself eating more to keep your blood glucose levels in the normal range, consult your health care provider about whether you need to adjust the amount of medication you take. Be sure to bring your blood glucose records with you so that he or she can see the patterns you've noticed.

blood glucose levels vary depending on the amount and types of food you eat, physical activity, and your stress level, for example, check blood glucose levels at different times of the day. A typical monitoring schedule might be to check your blood glucose when you get out of bed in the morning, before meals, and/or 1 to 2 hours after meals.

Ultimately, you'll begin to keep your blood glucose levels in a consistent range, but there will be times when you'll experience some highs and lows. Low blood glucose, or hypoglycemia, can occur if you're taking too much insulin or glucose-lowering medication, waiting too long to eat, skipping meals, exercising too much, drinking alcohol, or taking other medications which cause a drop in blood glucose levels. If your blood glucose falls below 80 mg./dl., and you're feeling shaky, sweaty, tired, hungry, and irritable and have a headache or blurred vision, test your blood glucose to determine if you need to eat something. If it's less than 80 mg./dl. and you have symptoms, or if it's below 70 mg./dl. and you don't have symptoms, eat a bread serving or drink 1/2 cup fruit juice or 1 cup milk. If you're unable to test your blood glucose and you're experiencing these symptoms, eat something with carbohydrates immediately.

On the other end of the spectrum, you could also have high blood glucose levels, called hyperglycemia. This happens when blood glucose levels are above normal, usually about 240 mg./dl. or higher, and stay there for a few days. When your blood glucose reaches these levels, it means your diabetes is not well controlled. High blood glucose levels can happen in hours or slowly over several days. The most common causes are not taking enough medication (insulin or glucose-lowering pills), eating too much food, emotional stress, infections, inactivity, and illness. If your blood glucose remains over 240 mg./dl. for several days, or if you're sick, you may need to test your urine ketones. A urine test (available from your pharmacy) will tell you if you have ketones in your urine. Your body makes ketones when your blood doesn't have enough insulin. Because ketones can make you very sick (vomiting, weakness, fast breathing, and a sweet smell on your breath), call your health care provider right away.

2. Hemoglobin A1c—Your Progress Report

Whereas monitoring blood glucose levels gives you a day-to-day indication of diabetes management, the hemoglobin A1c (glycosylated hemoglobin) test gives you a long-term progress report. It tells you whether your diabetes management plan has been effective for the past 2 to 3 months. It's a test that your health care provider performs at the clinic because he or she needs a sample of your blood. When you're keeping your blood glucose levels in the goal range of 70 to 150 mg./dl., your hemoglobin A1c test should be within the recommended range. If your blood glucose levels are not well controlled, your test results will be high. Visit your clinic two to four times each year to have the hemoglobin A1c test. Generally the normal value is in the range of 4 to 7 percent. Because this number varies slightly from clinic to clinic, you should ask your health care provider what your goal hemoglobin A1c should be.

3. Weight Checks

You might have noticed a theme—losing weight can improve your blood glucose levels and prevent chronic diseases associated with weight and diabetes. The good news is you can get these great health benefits from a weight loss of 10 to 20 pounds.

As you progress in your weight and diabetes management plan, it's helpful to track your weight on a regular basis. Ideally, you should weigh yourself no more than one time per week. The reason? Your weight can fluctuate as much as 3 to 5 pounds each day depending on how active you are, the number of beverages you drink, and what medications you take. If you're a woman, your weight varies with your menstrual cycle. Keep in mind, too, that the scale can't tell the difference between muscle and fat. Muscle weighs more than fat. So, if you have a muscular body type, you can expect to weigh more.

Additionally, as you increase activity, you may increase your muscle mass while decreasing your body fat. When this happens, you might not

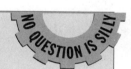

I've heard that apple-shaped people are at greater risk for heart disease and diabetes than pear-shaped people. Is that true?

Yes, it's true. People who have a waist that is larger around than their hips (apple shaped) are at greater risk for these diseases than people whose hips are larger than their waists (pear shaped). To determine your waist-to-hip ratio, measure your waist at the level of your belly button and measure your hips at the widest point. Then divide the waist number by the hip number. Men should aim for a number less than 1 and women less than 0.8. If your number is higher than this, you have an apple shape.

notice any difference in your scale weight even though you've probably lost inches. Yet the end result is the same—improved diabetes control. Try to avoid the daily weigh-in trap. Even if you're losing weight, it's hard to see a 1/4-pound weight loss on the scale. And when you don't, you may set yourself up to go off your program. Or if you do experience a decrease in weight, you may reward yourself detrimentally—for instance, by treating yourself to extra helpings of food.

4. Blood Lipids (Fats)

High cholesterol and triglyceride levels can contribute to cardiovascular (heart) disease. The steps to maintaining normal cholesterol and triglyceride levels are the same as your diabetes and weight management plan—lose weight, get active, and eat less fat. You'll learn more about how to eat less fat and change the types of fat you eat in chapter 10 and appendixes B and C. If you have high blood fat levels, cholesterol can build up in the walls of your arteries, leading to atherosclerosis—a form of heart disease. Eventually, the buildup can block off blood flow to the heart or brain, causing a heart attack or stroke.

Four blood fat numbers to monitor are total cholesterol, high-density lipoprotein (HDL), low-density lipoprotein (LDL), and triglycerides:

Total cholesterol gives you a general idea of how much cholesterol is circulating in your blood. Your target cholesterol level is less than 200 mg./dl.

LDL brings cholesterol into your system, clogging your arteries. Keep LDL below 130 mg./dl. or less than 100 mg./dl. if you've been diagnosed with heart disease.

HDL takes cholesterol out of the system, cleaning your arteries. Maintain your HDL above 35 mg./dl. if you're a man and above 45 mg./dl. if you're a woman. A high level of HDL (above 60 mg./dl.) is protective against heart disease.

Triglycerides are tiny packages of fat carried throughout your body to your fat cells. Once they arrive at your fat cells, insulin helps triglycerides enter the cell, allowing them to be stored as fat. When you have diabetes, you may not be able to store all the triglycerides because your insulin doesn't get the job done. This leads to high triglyceride levels, which may contribute to heart disease. Your goal triglyceride level is less than 200 mg./dl. or less than 150 mg./dl. if you already have heart disease.

5. Balancing Blood Pressure

High blood pressure, which occurs in more than 60 to 65 percent of people with diabetes, contributes to the development of heart disease, stroke, and other complications such as kidney disease. Blood pressure is the force generated by your heart as it pumps blood through your arteries to the rest of your body. Your blood pressure varies from one moment to the next depending on your activity level or emotional state. These fluctuations are normal. However, when your heart pushes blood too hard against the arteries, high blood pressure results.

Your goal is to keep your blood pressure less than 130/85. Have your blood pressure checked at least once a year. If it's high, talk with your health care provider about how exercise, weight loss, medication, and possibly a low-salt meal plan may improve your numbers.

Monitoring Your Progress

Tracking blood glucose, hemoglobin A1c, weight, blood lipids, and blood pressure will improve control of diabetes, help keep your weight in check, and manage your risk of long-term complications. But to do this, you need a monitoring system. Provided here are three methods to monitor your progress.

Because you may be checking blood glucose levels regularly, one option is to record them in a small notebook designed for people with diabetes or the memory program in your blood glucose monitor. A sample record is provided on page 60. These records help you and your health care provider assess your diabetes management. Remember to write down next to your blood glucose readings how you were feeling, any changes from your usual meal plan, and any physical activity you did during the day. Bring your record book with you when you visit your health care provider. These records help determine if you need to make changes in your glucose-lowering pills or insulin (if you take any) or in your meal plan.

For the health parameters you're monitoring every few months to once a year, track them with the following Know Your Numbers chart. Over time, using this chart will highlight for both you and your health care provider positive changes that have resulted from the lifestyle changes you've made. It will also identify areas that may need more attention.

Another tool you can use to monitor your diabetes care is the Take Charge: Your Checklist for Good Health form. If you're doing all of the

Know Your Numbers

TEST	GOAL RANGE	DATE:____	DATE:____	DATE:____
Hemoglobin A1c*	4% to 7%			
Weight				
Total cholesterol	Below 200			
HDL cholesterol	Above 35 (men) Above 45 (women)			
LDL cholesterol	Below 130			
Triglycerides	Below 200			
Blood pressure	Less than 130/85			

*Ask your doctor for your recommended hemoglobin A1c range.

action steps on the checklist, you're on target with your diabetes control and on the path to preventing or delaying long-term complications. If you aren't doing all the action steps, think about those you still need to do and how you can accomplish them.

You may even want to bring this checklist with you to each clinic visit to ask your health care provider if there are other measures you should take to manage your diabetes. Additionally, before each visit, remember to write out any questions you have about your medication, blood glucose levels, and so forth. Between visits, keep a list of any unusual symptoms you've experienced or concerns you want to discuss.

Take Charge: Your Checklist for Good Health

Read each statement and check "yes" for those action steps you are presently doing and "no" for those you have not yet achieved.

I check my blood glucose regularly and record it. Yes____ No____

My morning blood glucose is in the target range. Yes____ No____

My blood glucose levels during the day
    are in the target range. Yes____ No____

Each day I check my feet, looking for changes
    such as cuts and bruises. Yes____ No____

I eat at consistent meal and snack times. Yes____ No____

I monitor my portion sizes and eat similar
   amounts of food at each meal or snack. Yes___ No___

I get 30 minutes of physical activity each day. Yes___ No___

Every day I take my medication, if any,
   as prescribed by my doctor. Yes___ No___

I know my blood pressure and cholesterol numbers. Yes___ No___

I have my blood pressure checked at least once a year. Yes___ No___

If my cholesterol is high, I have it checked once a year. Yes___ No___

My weight is stable, or I am losing small amounts of weight
   at a rate no greater than 1/2 pound to 1 pound per week. Yes___ No___

I have a yearly physical exam with my health care provider. Yes___ No___

Every year I have a dilated eye examination. Yes___ No___

Bringing It All Together

Your overall goal is improved blood glucose management. Yet by monitoring weight, blood fats, and blood pressure, for example, you can prevent or delay long-term complications associated with diabetes. The key is monitoring your progress regularly to assess how you're doing, staying on track with your diabetes and weight management plan, and making changes in your care plan as appropriate.

Blood Glucose Record

WEEK OF: _____

TARGET BLOOD GLUCOSE: _____ **AVER. WEEKLY BLOOD GLUCOSE:** _____

	BREAKFAST	LUNCH	DINNER	SNACK
MONDAY Before				
After				
Medication				
Comments:				
TUESDAY Before				
After				
Medication				
Comments:				
WEDNESDAY Before				
After				
Medication				
Comments:				
THURSDAY Before				
After				
Medication				
Comments:				
FRIDAY Before				
After				
Medication				
Comments:				
SATURDAY Before				
After				
Medication				
Comments:				
SUNDAY Before				
After				
Medication				
Comments:				

Reprinted with permission from HealthCheques. Blood Glucose Record developed by RD Concepts, 1997. P.O. Box 47651, Minneapolis, MN 55447.

setting goals within reach

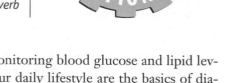

> The journey of a thousand miles
> starts with a single step.
> *Chinese proverb*

Building healthier eating habits, monitoring blood glucose and lipid levels, and adding more activity to your daily lifestyle are the basics of diabetes control and weight management. But how do you combine them into a comprehensive, personalized health plan? By setting goals.

There are three different types of goals: long-term, short-term, and weekly goals, or, as they're called here, **weekly action steps.** A long-term goal identifies what you hope to accomplish in the long run, whether it's weight loss or improved diabetes control. The biggest issue in setting a long-term goal is making sure it's realistic. Short-term goals are checkpoints along the way for you to assess whether you're on track to reaching your long-term goal. Although it's important to know the big picture you want to achieve, your focus for diabetes and weight management is on weekly action steps. These are the gradual changes you'll make in your lifestyle habits on a daily and weekly basis to positively impact your health.

By the end of this chapter, you'll not only have established your personal long-term goal for weight loss and diabetes control but have mapped out your way there by getting started with weekly action steps.

Why Set Goals?

Several years ago, a study was done to determine what top executives of Fortune 500 companies had in common. Was it an MBA degree from Harvard? Inheritance of money or a business from a relative? Diversification of their assets? Actually, none of these were correct. All the executives had, at some time in their career, identified and written down their long- and short-term goals. The moral of this story is not how to become an executive of a major company, but how important writing down the specific goals you want to achieve is toward success.

But this first step can be difficult. The fear of failure and demands on your time can prevent you from establishing goals. Although there are many barriers to success, the following five can seriously deter you from setting goals for better health:

1. Superman or Superwoman complex. In today's society many people believe they have to be able to do it all—have a successful, satisfying career, raise a happy family, and be involved in the community. The list goes on and on. But to reach your goals, you have to be realistic about your time and the demands in your life.

2. Personal disorganization. Disorganization steals your time. Whether in your personal or professional life, if you don't have a clear picture of what needs to get done and by when, you're less efficient. Getting organized gives you time to work on things that top your priority list.

3. Fear of saying no. As you begin the journey of weight and diabetes management, acknowledge that your health is a top priority. Other things will have to take a backseat so that you can take care of your health.

4. Lack of self-discipline. You may find that you've been putting off getting serious about weight loss. Take charge of your health instead of waiting for someone else to do it for you (because they won't).

NO QUESTION IS SILLY

I haven't gotten comfortable with when or how often I should reward myself. Any suggestions?

The purpose of rewards is to acknowledge positive changes you've made and to motivate yourself to stick with your weekly action steps. In all areas of your life, behaviors that are rewarded are more likely to be repeated, so periodically treating you to something you enjoy will strengthen new habits you've built. There is no specific time frame that you have to follow for rewards. If you've been struggling with an action step and finally tackle it, reward yourself. If you achieve 90 percent of your weekly action steps for the month, find a way to celebrate. The important thing is to build rewards in to your weight and diabetes management plan.

5. Procrastination. Lack of confidence about the end result, fear of making a mistake, and perfectionism can all lead to procrastination. Before you set your goals, admit there is a risk involved. Tackling easy tasks before unpleasant ones is a natural tendency, but one to avoid as you set health goals.

As you move into the goal-setting process, consider and deal with the factors that may affect your own comfort level when setting personal goals.

Getting to It

The work sheet on page 66 walks you through the steps of setting your personal health goals. The first step is to develop your long-term goal. Although there's no specific time frame you have to meet, try to set a goal you'd like to achieve at least one year from today. Your goal should be personal, reflecting your own wants and health needs. Don't let someone else—your doctor or spouse—overinfluence your goals. You're the one who must be committed to achieving them. If you're setting a long-term goal related to weight loss, refer back to the section in chapter 2 on reasonable weight loss goals.

The following are some examples of long-term goals:

I will lose weight to manage my diabetes and to reduce or eliminate my diabetes medication.

I will work to maintain a normal hemoglobin A1c level to prevent the possible complications of diabetes.

I will establish healthful eating and lifestyle habits to manage diabetes and my weight, and to feel great.

Over the next 5 years, I'll lose 20 pounds and keep it off.

I will adopt healthier habits to lower my cholesterol level by 10 percent over the next year.

Once you've chosen a long-term health goal that fits your lifestyle, begin breaking it down into manageable pieces by setting short-term goals and time frames. For example, if your goal is to lose weight, your first short-term goal may be to lose 10 pounds in the next year. If your goal is to normalize your hemoglobin A1c, your first short-term goal may be to routinely monitor blood glucose for the next 3 months. Give yourself a realistic amount of time for these goals, as suggested in the examples.

To get started, read through the example on the next page and then use the work sheet to set your personal goals. Take time to do this activity; avoid the temptation to procrastinate. Setting goals is an essential step on your route to success in weight management and diabetes control.

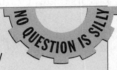

After setting my goals, I realized how personal they are. My husband asked to see them, but I don't know if I'm comfortable sharing them. Do I have to show others my goals?

Goals are very personal, especially when they relate to your health. Whether to share them is really your decision. One thing to consider, however, is that support from other people can be crucial to your success. You want to share your goals with the people who will have some responsibility in helping you attain them. For example, if you have decided to focus on limiting fat as a goal, but are not the person primarily responsible for grocery shopping, it may be difficult to reach this goal. In this situation, it would be beneficial and less frustrating to share this goal with the person who does most of the shopping. This doesn't mean that you have to share all your goals, only the parts that pertain to others.

Go for the Goals *Example*

By setting the following goals, I am taking control of my health and well-being.

1. My long-term health goal is:

To develop healthful eating and lifestyle habits to manage diabetes and my weight, and to feel great!

2. Short-term goals to reach this long-term goal: Time frame:

Assess current meal patterns and daily fat intake.   *May 15*

Reduce fat intake to 30% of calories from fat.   *August 1*

Increase activity to 30 minutes per day,   *October 15*
      6 days a week.

Maintain weight through holiday season.   *January 1*

Work on stress management.   *March 15*

3. Personal strengths and attributes that will enable me to reach these goals:

Good time management skills.

I'm creative—a skill I can use in modifying recipes
      to be lower in fat.

I'm very motivated to make lifestyle changes for
      improved diabetes control.

I'm a morning person, so I'll be able to get active
      before I leave for work.

Go for the Goals

By setting the following goals, I am taking control of
my health and well-being.

1. My long-term health goal is:

_____

_____

_____

2. Short-term goals to reach this long-term goal: Time frame:

_____

_____

_____

_____

_____

_____

_____

_____

3. Personal strengths and attributes that will enable me to reach these goals:

_____

_____

_____

_____

_____

_____

_____

_____

_____

Tips for Effective Goal Setting

Use the following questions to assess the goals you've just set.

Are they realistic? It may be tempting to set easy goals to guarantee your own success, but in the end neither you nor your health will benefit. On the other hand, setting goals that go beyond the time, resources, and abilities you have is self-defeating. Using words such as "I'll never," "I'll always," or "I must" suggests your goals may not be appropriate. Realistic goals leave open the opportunity for success as well as the possibility of failure.

Are they flexible? In the real world, things change. You could suddenly have an ill parent who demands your attention, need to look for a new job because your current one is being eliminated, or find yourself promoted from assistant to head Little League coach as your predecessor moves out of town. To fit into the ups and downs of life, your short-term goals need to be flexible. Build in weeks where your goal is to maintain, not lose, weight. Don't force yourself to exercise when you have a sinus infection and should be resting. If your legs are just too tired to run that last half mile, walk it instead.

Are they positive? In today's society, it's more common to be negative about yourself than positive. How often do you go to a dinner party and talk about what a great job you're doing at work, how well you're raising your kids, or how excited you are about the weight loss you've achieved? Yet to set yourself up for success rather than failure, it's essential to use positive statements in setting your goals. Can you see the difference between "I'll stop eating so many doughnuts" and "When I crave something sweet, I'll make low-fat choices?"

Are they specific and easy to measure? Lofty, ambiguous goals are not effective. Goals need to be well defined and as specific as possible. They should state exactly what behavior you'll change. "I want to lose some weight" is very nonspecific. "I will improve my eating and physical activity habits over the next year to lose 10 pounds and gain control of my diabetes." Now that's a specific goal! As well as being specific, it's measurable (to lose 10 pounds) and provides you with a time frame to track your progress.

Are they visual? Writing goals and hiding them in the middle of this book is neat and orderly, but not effective. Keep your goals in front of you and visual, so that they continue to be your priority. You could write them in your daily planner, post them on your bathroom mirror, or tape them in the center of your car steering wheel. Find a spot that keeps your goals close at hand.

Are there built-in rewards? When behaviors are rewarded, they're more likely to be repeated. So with all your goals—both long- and short-term—develop your own reward system. When considering rewards, make sure they're of personal value. Try a new tie, an outfit of a color you never felt comfortable in before, a weekend getaway, season tickets for a local sports team, a new exercise video, or a manicure. Because it's one of the areas you are working to gain control over, avoid using food as a reward. A common question is how often you should reward yourself. This is for you to decide, but consider logical weight reductions such as every five pounds, drops in hemoglobin A1c levels, or time frames of having maintained new habits such as being physically active consistently for eight weeks. You want to make the reward something to work toward and look forward to.

If, after reviewing your goals against these six questions, you find some changes you'd like to make, go back and do so. Remember, goals can be effective only if they reflect your personal needs and lifestyle. As you move forward through the process of managing weight to improve diabetes control, you will frequently come back to these goals. So, before you move on,

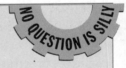

Long-term goals, short-term goals, action steps—I'm getting confused and overwhelmed. Can't I just set one goal and work on it?

That depends on whether your one goal is a long-term goal or more of a weekly action step. A long-term goal will set the direction for the health results you want to achieve. Are you after better diabetes control? Weight loss? A lowered risk of heart disease and the other complications of diabetes? Although it's important to set long- and short-term goals, you don't need to think about them that often. Refer back to them every couple of months as a progress check. You want to put most of your energy, concentration, and focus into your weekly action steps. What are the habits and behaviors you want to work on to achieve better health? Consistent meal patterns? Choosing lower-fat snacks? Adding 30 minutes of physical activity every day? The Take Action Today tips on pages 70 to 72 are examples of how specific and action oriented your weekly steps should be. Set between one and three very specific action steps that you will work on each week.

be sure that you're comfortable with them and feel positive about the direction you've chosen.

Weekly Action Steps

The final step in goal setting is ongoing, and where the fun really begins. To set up weekly action steps, you now need to break your short-term goals down into even smaller increments. By setting many small steps in the upcoming weeks, you'll find that these small steps will add up to giant leaps toward meeting your long-term goal.

Weekly action steps should be very specific. If you want to identify the sources of fat in your current eating plan, your first weekly action step may be to purchase a book listing the fat content of various foods. Your action step for the following week could be to track what you ate for breakfast for three days and calculate the fat grams in these meals. These measurable, action-oriented steps will help you keep a forward momentum going.

People are often initially skeptical about weekly action steps. You may be asking yourself right now, "If my diabetes is serious enough, shouldn't I be trying to change as much as I can as soon as possible?" Although there are various changes you could make today that would benefit your health, you could be overwhelmed (and end up giving up on making any changes) if you try to do too much too soon. Long-term weight and diabetes management is what you're after, and gradual changes you can incorporate into your daily routine are the best way to achieve it.

Weekly action steps work for three reasons. First, they allow you to work on one thing at a time. By breaking down more cumbersome objectives into practical, measurable actions, you can fit these steps into your lifestyle. Second, they prevent you from getting overwhelmed by the larger and seemingly difficult short-term goals you've set. Gradual changes are easier to accept. Third, weekly action steps work because after weeks of taking these actions, you'll discover that you have actually achieved some of your short-term goals and are well on your way to reaching your long-term goal. Success will have snuck up on you.

Perhaps the most important factor to consider when you set weekly action steps is to make them very specific, targeted actions. To get you started, this chapter provides Take Action Today tips in four areas crucial to weight and diabetes management: physical activity, low-fat eating, portion control, and lifestyle habits. Don't feel compelled to use all or any of these tips. If you're more comfortable using your own action steps, do so. If in the weeks ahead you find yourself struggling for weekly steps, refer back to this listing for more ideas to keep you moving on the road to success. Although they are called weekly action steps, it's OK to work on some for a longer time if they're particularly challenging behaviors. Then move on to a new action step. Remember—building habits is an ongoing, step-by-step process. In the chapters that follow, you'll find **Take Action Today tips** on topics ranging from support to stress management to holiday eating. Consider using these as your weekly action steps as you work through your own weight and diabetes management issues.

The Take Action, Make It Happen chart that follows these tips is provided for your use in tracking weekly action steps, assessing progress, and setting reward time frames in the weeks and months ahead.

Physical Activity

This weekend I will participate in a family bike trip.

Two days this week, I will park my car in the spot farthest from the door at work.

I will find a partner to walk with during lunch 1 day this week.

While watching TV, I will do stretching exercises during the commercials.

I will call the local shopping mall to get information on their walking program.

Instead of taking the car, I'll walk on two local errands (renting a video, picking up milk, etc.).

I'll price exercise bikes at three stores this week.

I will lift weights 2 nights this week.

I'll enter the racquetball tournament at the club this weekend.

I will set the alarm clock 1 hour early and exercise before work twice this week.

I will walk the dog 2 nights this week.

I'll cut the lawn with the push mower instead of using the riding mower.

I will shovel the driveway instead of using the snowblower.

I'll invest in a good pair of walking shoes.

I will take the stairs instead of the elevator at least three times this week.

Low-Fat Eating

I will try one new low-fat recipe.

I'll skip the popcorn and candy when I go to a movie this weekend.

For my business trip, I'll call the airline ahead of time and order a low-fat meal for the flight.

I'll use the shopping list provided in appendix B to avoid impulse purchases when I grocery shop this week.

I will eat 1 fruit serving at breakfast 4 days this week.

I will eat a nonmeat entrée at least once this week.

I'll bring a healthful lunch to work 2 to 3 times this week instead of eating out.

I will buy two new low-fat products during my regular grocery shopping trip.

I will try a low-fat sandwich when I visit a fast-food restaurant this week.

On Sunday, I will cut up raw vegetables to have accessible for snacking during the week.

I'll purchase low-fat snacks to keep in my "emergency food drawer" at work.

I'll make recipe modifications to lower the fat in one of my family's favorite recipes (see appendix C to learn how).

I will bring a low-fat item to the potluck at work.

I'll count my daily fat grams every other day this week.

Portion Control

One day this week, I will measure out all the food I eat.

When I eat out Friday night, I will ask for a take-home carton, and when my meal comes, I'll put half the portion in it immediately or share my meal with a friend.

During my two business luncheons, I'll stop eating when I'm 80 percent full (satisfied, not stuffed).

I will use the smallest bowls, plates, and utensils I have at home.

At the holiday buffet (or all-you-can-eat buffet luncheon or dinner), I'll visit the buffet line only once.

I will limit my cookie consumption to two, even if they are fat free.

At dinner 4 nights, I'll leave several bites of food on my plate.

On 3 consecutive days, I will eat consistent portions and types of food at each meal.

I will purchase single servings of healthful foods (pretzels, low-fat cookies, or crackers) to have available for snacks.

I will order a small, instead of a medium, pizza on bowling night.

Lifestyle Habits

During at least one bout of anger or frustration this week, I'll write in my journal instead of eating.

I will develop a list of 10 things I can do instead of eating when I'm bored, angry, or depressed.

Three nights this week, I will eat dinner at the table instead of in front of the TV.

Three days this week, I will take an hour just for myself—to read a book, take a bath, play a computer game, or catch a catnap.

I will plan to get 8 hours of sleep at least 5 nights this week.

I will join a golf or bowling league this week.

I will eat dinner at the same time 5 nights this week.

I will write a positive statement about myself every day.

Take Action, Make It Happen

Set one to three action steps each week. Reward yourself once a month or as often as you feel you've made progress in changing behaviors.

WEEK	WEEKLY ACTION STEP	ACHIEVED?
One	On Sunday I'll cut up vegetables to have for snacking all week.	yes

REWARD

To record additional weeks, photocopy this page.

Take Action, Make It Happen

Set one to three action steps each week. Reward yourself once a month or as often as you feel you've made progress in changing behaviors.

WEEKLY ACTION STEP   **ACHIEVED?**

_____

_____

_____

_____

_____

_____

_____

_____

_____

_____

_____

_____

_____

_____

_____

_____

_____

_____

REWARD

_____

To record additional weeks, photocopy this page.

relinking
THE BEHAVIOR CHAIN

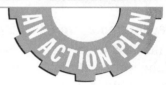

> The ultimate measure of a man is not
> where he stands in moments of comfort
> and convenience, but where he stands
> at times of challenge and controversy.
> *Martin Luther King Jr.*

Gradual changes such as eating lunch at the same time each day, keeping low-fat snack foods in your desk drawer, or walking the dog a few times each week may seem like small steps, but they make a big difference in your health and well-being. By changing your actions on a daily and weekly basis, you can begin to see changes in health parameters such as blood glucose and cholesterol levels or your weight.

Once you've gone through the process of setting goals, you have a clearer picture of what you want to accomplish and the specific changes you need to make in upcoming months. Now it's time for the *how*—how to eat differently, how to be consistent about physical activity, and how to replace old habits with new, healthier ones. In this chapter, you'll examine your readiness to change various lifestyle habits, learn the how of changing behaviors, and, in the end, gain the skills you need to achieve the health goals you've set for yourself.

The Stages of Change

You might have a good idea of some of the changes you need to make to improve your health, but you probably haven't assessed whether you're really ready to change each of these behaviors. Take, for example, action steps that have been used over the past several weeks. When it comes to action steps set for physical activity, you may always be marking a "yes" in the "achieved" column on the Take Action, Make It Happen work sheet from chapter 6. But when it comes to action steps for blood glucose monitoring, your "achieved" rate may be up and down, with more downs than ups. Although you might be getting frustrated by this type of track record, don't get discouraged. What you've realized, without even knowing it, is that you may be more ready to change some behaviors and less ready to change others. It's normal to progress through different behavior changes at various rates. By understanding your readiness to change, you can set more appropriate action steps for different behaviors. To begin this process, become familiar with the five stages of change.

Precontemplation (Why Should I Change?)

In this first stage, you don't see any reason to alter your behaviors. You might feel comfortable with your weight partially because it hasn't adversely affected your health yet. Work, family, or other activities may be your current focus. It's an unfortunate truth that comfort and general satisfaction with your current life situation rarely motivate change.

Contemplation (I Guess This Is Real)

This is where it hits. All in one visit, your doctor diagnoses you with Type II diabetes and tells you to lose weight. You see a nurse, spend an hour with a dietitian, and go home with a handful of brochures describing your new lifestyle. In 4 hours your entire life has changed. "Ugh," you scream, "I have diabetes. Can't I die from diabetes?"

That's when reality and your own life expectancy sink in. Now you've arrived at contemplation. You realize that you need to make some new choices; after all, your life, health, and well-being depend on it. In the weeks and months following diagnosis, you think about making some changes. You're well intentioned but haven't developed a realistic plan of action.

Preparation (I Think I Can Do This)

At this midpoint, you could go either way, forward into action, or backward into contemplation. You're committed and motivated but need more determination to really affect your behavior. You make plans to walk 2 miles before going to work but hit the snooze button when the alarm sounds. You count fat grams at home but don't factor in your business luncheon. You've set a long-term health goal but haven't started using action steps. You're still unsure of exactly how to make positive changes.

Action (I'm Doing It)

Ready, set, go. You've gotten ready, you've set the stage, and you're off and running. Well, not necessarily running. Maybe walking, or biking, or aerobicizing. Or eating more fruits and vegetables and fewer high-fat snacks. The point is that when you've reached this stage of change, you're taking action steps to adopt a healthier lifestyle and build a new you. You've found the motivation, commitment, time, and energy to put your health first.

Maintenance (It's Second Nature)

This stage of change lasts the longest—hopefully a lifetime. Once you reach your health goals, you'll initially find that maintaining your new behaviors takes a conscious effort. With repetition over time, these behaviors become routine. When you no longer need to think of them at all, they have truly become habits. If you've maintained a new habit for at least six months, you've reached this stage of change for that behavior. But remember, change is a process. Even in maintenance, you'll probably experience occasional lapses or slips (see chapter 13). This is inevitable. The key is to pick up where you left off and continue your new, healthier habits.

It's probably more obvious now that you can be in one stage of change with one behavior and a different stage of change with another behavior. For instance, physical activity may come easy (the "maintenance" stage), while blood glucose monitoring may be only in the "preparation" stage because action steps are often not completed.

Use the following Make the Change work sheet to examine your weekly action steps. First, list the action steps you've been setting over the past several weeks. Next, determine your stage of change for each action based on the descriptions given. The behaviors for which you are in the preparation or action stage are ones you're really ready to change, and they should be your focus. If you find you're in the precontemplation or contemplation stage for other behaviors, use the work sheet and set new action steps that are within your current mind-set. For behaviors in the precontemplation stage, weigh the pros and cons for you personally in making this change. Gather more information. Figure out where the resistance to change is coming from. To work on behaviors in the contemplation stage, discover what it will take to motivate you to move toward action. Talk to others who have been in a similar situation. Working through a particular stage of change may lead you from one stage into the next and then into action, where you'll really notice changes in your behavior.

Make the Change Work Sheet

1. List action steps that you've set over the past several weeks.

Stage of Change

example: I'll carry my lunch to work 3 days this week.   preparation

2. For action steps in precontemplation or contemplation, list two appropriate action steps for the particular stage of change.

Action Step 1: I'll carry my lunch to work 3 days this week.

Revised Action Step: I'll make a list of 10 benefits of carrying my lunch to work.

At the store, I'll buy frozen entrées for work lunches.

Action Step 2:

Revised Action Step:

Action Step 3:

Revised Action Step:

The Behavior Chain

Now that you've identified the behaviors you're ready to change, you'll learn how to change them. You can gain skill in replacing old habits with new, healthier ones by looking into the behavior chain of your current habits. Most behaviors are learned, and they follow a cycle or pattern. When you get up in the morning, do you brush your teeth first or get right into the shower? What is the last thing you do before you leave the house for work every day? Do you always mow the lawn in the same pattern? On the same day of the week?

These behaviors are not inborn or imprinted on your brain from the start of your life. They're habits. Because you've done them the same way again and again, you no longer think about these actions and how you do them. They're learned behaviors, and you operate on automatic pilot when doing them.

If you sat down and wrote out the individual steps involved with these behaviors, you'd see that the sequence of events is always the same. For example, say you're on the way out the door to work. Here's the chain of events leading up to your departure: let dog out → pack lunch into work bag → put coat on → find car keys → leave house → get to work on time → sigh with relief because the day has started well.

As you can see, there's a chain of linked actions leading up to actually leaving the house. These steps are likely to be the same each day. This behavior chain can also be applied to any health behavior or action. Consider the following health behavior chain: missed lunch → hungry on

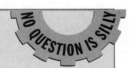

I get so overwhelmed when I think about the big project of changing behaviors that I never even start. How can I get beyond this?

In changing any behavior, the key is to take it one step at a time, and this is why weekly action steps work so well. Choose one behavior to change first. Work at analyzing the behavior and identifying how to change it to a healthier outcome. Set one weekly action step for this behavior. See how this feels and then do it again. Avoid the temptation to do too much at once. Set action steps for one week at a time and don't look beyond this time frame. Soon you'll have many individual weeks of successfully doing the new behavior, and it will become a habit. Small successes over time give big results, yet won't overwhelm you.

drive home from work → see fast-food restaurant → french fries, large burger, and shake sound quick, easy, and appetizing → order meal through drive through → eat while driving rest of way home → too full to eat healthful meal planned for dinner → feel guilty that you ate junk food.

What did you learn after examining this behavior chain? The benefit of looking at these chains is that they help identify the specific events that lead up to the behavior. If you hadn't missed lunch, you most likely wouldn't have been so hungry on the drive home from work. If the fast-food restaurant wasn't on your route home, you wouldn't have stopped and ordered foods not planned for in that day's meal plan.

Once the chain is identified, you can determine where the weak links are in the chain and make changes to affect the end result—the sabotaging behavior. Use the foregoing example in the following exercise. Considering this scenario, list two places where you see weak links in the chain.

1. _____
2. _____

Now, identify how these weak links could be broken and relinked to build new, healthier habits.

1. _____
2. _____

This chain could easily be broken at any of the five first links. Potential chain relinkings for a healthier lifestyle include

keeping healthful snacks in the car to curb hunger on the ride home from work,

changing the route home to avoid the fast-food restaurant,

ordering something healthful from the fast-food menu,

ordering something small from the menu—just enough to satisfy your hunger until you get home.

As you review behavior chains, you'll find that each link falls into one of the following three aspects of behavior:

Antecedents are the events, situations, or feelings that lead up to the action. In the example, missing lunch and seeing the fast-food restaurant are the antecedents.

Behaviors are the actions themselves. In the example, eating the fast food is the behavior.

Consequences happen after the action. Most often the behavior leads to feelings and attitudes about the behavior or yourself. Here the key consequence is the guilt felt after eating the fast-food meal. The consequences that result from any behavior can determine if that behavior is repeated or not. Take these three aspects of behavior one step further. As you examined the example behavior chain to determine where it could be broken and relinked for healthier behaviors, it became obvious that the break needs to come before the action happens. Antecedents are the logical place for the breaks to occur. The earlier the chain is broken, often the more successful you'll be at effectively changing behaviors.

Now that you've thoroughly examined the chain, it's time to get personal. Use the following Break the Chain Activity page to detail the antecedents, behaviors, and consequences of your own behavior chains. Before you start, think of one specific behavior you'd like to change, such as watching television in the evening instead of exercising, canceling doctor's appointments, or not making healthful choices at business lunches. Then follow through the steps in the activity. Refer back to these pages after you've positively changed this behavior and are ready to tackle others. Remember, behavior change is a process. Success comes by taking one behavior at a time and relinking its chain, rather than by trying to tackle several behaviors at the same time.

One of the behaviors I'd like to work on would involve some changes by my family as well. How do I handle this?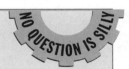

Chapter 8 deals with the whole issue of support during weight control and diabetes management, but in the meantime there are some things you can do. Plan a family meeting so that everyone has a chance to ask questions about diabetes and so that you can explain the changes that you're about to make. Be clear with your family on how this may affect them and let them know how important their support is to you. You may even want to suggest that this would be a great time for the entire family to start building healthier lifestyle habits. Everyone's health would benefit, and you'd make changes together, creating a very supportive network.

Break the Chain Activity

Behavior I will change: _____

_____

_____

Behavior chain leading to this behavior: _____

_____

_____

_____

_____

_____

_____

Antecedents: _____

Behavior: _____

_____

Consequences: _____

Weakest links in my chain: _____

How I will break these weak links
and relink them to build a healthier habit: _____

_____

Healthier habit that will result: _____

_____

_____

Days chain break attempted: _____

Successfully relinked chain? Yes _____ No _____

Reward to myself for building this healthier habit: _____

_____

_____

Food Triggers

When you completed the Break the Chain Activity, it's likely that one of the behaviors you examined was related to food and possibly involved eating for reasons other than hunger. In the United States, people haven't been trained to eat only when their bodies tell them they're hungry. People eat at noon because that's lunchtime. Many couples eat two big meals on holidays because they visit both sides of the family. Spectators eat at a football game because everyone else does. After a confrontation at work, people eat a candy bar to deal with the frustration.

For many people, a key issue in weight and diabetes management is learning to deal with these food triggers and breaking the chain that leads to this behavior. To explore things that trigger you to overeat and learn how to break this behavior chain, take the following Triggers That Trip You Up quiz.

Triggers That Trip You Up

1. Check all the following that apply to you or where you find yourself overeating or craving certain foods.

A _____ When I walk by a bakery, I am lured inside by the smell of fresh-baked pastries.

B _____ My department at work is having a potluck lunch, and I can't resist trying everything.

C _____ When I head to the movie theater on a rainy day, I treat myself to popcorn and candy.

D _____ When I get together with old friends, I suggest we meet for dinner.

E _____ After an argument with my spouse or significant other, I can tunnel through a pint of ice cream.

A _____ The box of cookies sitting out on the counter top calls to me every time I walk by.

B _____ A Caribbean cruise makes indulging an exotic must.

C _____ At a baseball game, I usually order a hot dog, even though I had dinner before the game.

D _____ When my coworkers order pizza, I join them for a slice or two without thinking about whether I'm hungry or not.

E _____ During 2 days of waiting to hear about a possible promotion, I frequently find my hand in the candy dish.

continued on next page

Triggers That Trip You Up (continued)

A_____ The local restaurant displays its world-famous cakes and cheesecakes in the front window, and I can't walk by without having a piece.

B _____ I decide to throw caution (and healthy eating) to the winds for my sister's 50th birthday party on Saturday night.

C _____ What's a road trip without sugar in the forms of soda pop and candy?

D _____ A coworker and I work late. I suggest coffee and dessert to call it a night.

E _____ My best friend just canceled our plans for the third Saturday night in a row. Maybe chocolate ice cream will step in as a substitute friend.

A _____ The Dairy Queen commercial forces me to my car and down the road for an ice cream treat.

B _____ I love Thanksgiving and can't get enough of the special foods that come only once a year.

C _____ My Tuesday-night ritual is 2 hours of sitcoms and a bag of chips.

D _____ When I make plans with Bob, it's always the same thing—beers, burgers, and fries at the nightlife hot spot.

E _____ I feel fat, so I must be fat. I may as well eat.

A _____ Chocolate—just the word itself makes my mouth water.

B _____ What's a weekend getaway to the lake without bratwurst, hot dogs, and s'mores.

C _____ After the play-by-play of the Super Bowl, I can give a play-by-play on the taste of all the snacks served at the Super Bowl party.

D _____ Happy hour wouldn't be happy if my friends and I didn't graze our way through the appetizer menu.

E _____ Eating seems to fill the time when boredom strikes.

2. Total up the number of checks in each of the following categories:

A	C	E
B	D	

3. What you'll find is that one (or maybe two) of the areas have the highest score, corresponding to the following food triggers:

A Sensory Triggers. You respond to the sight or smell of food.

B Special Event Triggers. Vacations, parties, and holidays are situations in which you tend to overeat.

C Activity Triggers. You associate eating with certain activities, such as sporting events, movies, and watching television.

Triggers That Trip You Up (continued)

D People Triggers. You tend to plan social activities around eating events. Watching other people eat prompts you to eat.

E Emotional Triggers. Whether it was a bad day at work or you're feeling lonely or bored, you eat in response to your emotions.

So which triggers apply to you? Although you may not have recognized them before, taking this quiz can make your overeating triggers glaringly obvious. Now that you've identified what situations, events, or emotions trigger the overeating, you have two options. First you can take a particular trigger situation and walk through the Break the Chain Activity. Learn where the weak links are in your chain and relink it to be a healthier trigger. Train yourself so that the smell of a bakery sends you off running (literally) in the other direction. The second option is to find one or more of the following suggestions that will help you deal with your food triggers and use them as action steps in upcoming weeks.

Tips for Combating Food Triggers

Combatting Sensory Triggers

Keep tempting food in opaque containers at home. Out of sight, out of mind.

Dish out a normal portion of tempting foods. Freeze the rest.

Turn off the television during commercials or become a channel surfer—find a channel not showing commercials.

Wait it out. After 20 minutes, your craving will typically pass.

Allow yourself to go in and buy a fresh-baked loaf of bread or other healthful option instead of a cookie or pastry when walking by a bakery.

Change routes you usually drive to avoid fast-food restaurants and other food shops that tempt you.

Combatting Special Event Triggers

Bring a healthful food item when attending a potluck so that you know you'll have something nutritious to eat.

Choose a cruise or resort vacation that caters to the health conscious.

Host a party so that you can control the menu.

Eat a healthful snack before going to a party so that you're not starved when you arrive.

Plan what you will eat at the special event before going.

Position yourself at parties at the opposite end of the buffet or hors d'oeuvres table.

Keep a low-calorie drink in your hand at parties. It's more difficult to snack with just one hand.

Use the smallest plate available at a buffet or potluck.

Combatting Activity Triggers

Do leg lifts, walk in place, or lift weights while watching television.

Take up crocheting, knitting, woodworking, crossword puzzles, or another hobby to occupy your hands while watching television.

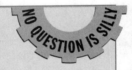

My problem with losing weight has always been continuing the new habits I've built and being consistent. Any suggestions?

An important thing to consider is the type of person you are. Are you a planner? If so, schedule time for weekly meal planning and make an appointment to exercise. Are you very outgoing and need other people involved? Then find an exercise partner or a personal trainer or a friend who is also interested in losing weight. Do you have a full-time job, a family, and little quality time for yourself? For your lifestyle, find the healthiest items on the local takeout menu, work out during your lunch hour, or swap baby-sitting time with friends to make time for activity. The key is to make your new, healthier behaviors a part of your everyday routine, no matter what your personal style.

Choose a low-fat food item such as a soft pretzel, frozen yogurt, or grilled chicken sandwich at sporting events.

Arrive at the movie theater just as the movie is scheduled to start. You'll be rushed to find a seat, leaving no time to purchase treats.

Before going, visualize yourself successfully attending a sporting event and maintaining your meal plan. How do you feel? Keep these thoughts in mind when you actually go to the event.

Combatting People Triggers

Do an activity that still allows socializing when planning get-togethers with friends. In-line skating, golfing, bowling, a walk on the shore, window shopping at the mall, or a trip to the local zoo gets you moving yet allows for catching up.

Before you go, set a time limit for happy hour and similar events. Make sure the time limit allows enough time for socializing but expires before other people's appetizer orders tempt you to make choices not within your meal plan.

Turn your usual "pig out" friend into a healthy-habit friend. Perhaps he or she wants to build healthier habits, too, and your Tuesday nights can become racquetball or tennis competitions.

Let those close to you know you're trying to lose weight and how they can avoid tempting you.

Combatting Emotional Triggers

Write a list of 10 ways to deal with emotions that are not related to food. Keep this list handy and refer to it when you need to.

Tackle your emotions head-on. Dealing with the emotion immediately, whether it involves confronting a coworker, discussing an unpleasant topic with your spouse, or disciplining a child, will release the emotion and your urge to eat.

Exercise. It's a great way to release stress and many other emotions.

Purchase a relaxation tape and use it, instead of food, to deal with stressful situations.

Call or write a near and dear friend.

I'm halfway through this book and haven't lost even a pound. I'm frustrated and feel as if this program is just another scam.

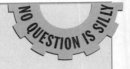

First, rethink your expectations. Once you decided you needed to lose weight, did you expect it to come off in a month? For permanent weight loss, a gradual weight loss is best—not more than 1/2 pound to 1 pound per week. Also, consider how long it took you to gain weight. Flip through the month pages in a calendar as a visual reminder of how long it took you to reach your current weight. It's not realistic to expect weight to come off in a month when it took months, if not years, to gain it.

Second, instead of focusing on the number on the scale, think about all the positive strides you've made in changing behaviors. If you're being more physically active, choosing lower-fat foods, or monitoring your blood glucose more consistently than before, it's important to acknowledge these new habits. Changing habits you've had for years isn't simple, and the fact that you've built new behaviors has much significance for your health. These changes may have led to reductions in your cholesterol, blood pressure, or glycosylated-hemoglobin level. If you haven't had these levels checked in a while, make an appointment to do so. You might be pleasantly surprised with the results.

Third, remember that muscle weighs more than fat. If you've become more physically active, you could be losing fat and gaining muscle. Even though the number on the scale hasn't changed, your body composition and shape may have (you've lost inches, not pounds).

teaming up for support

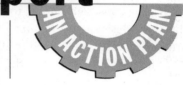

A true friend unbosoms freely, advises justly, assists readily, adventures boldly, takes all patiently, defends courageously, and continues a friend unchangeably.
William Penn

Think back to when you learned to ride a bike. If you were like most kids, you probably started with training wheels. The tiny tires supported your bicycle while you learned the art of balancing while pedaling. Each day you rode, your balance got a little better. Soon you felt ready—or at least more confident in your ability—to ride without the extra support, and your parents took off the training wheels.

Your diabetes and weight management program is similar to learning how to ride a bike. Initially you need to train yourself how to build lifestyle habits. Because this takes an investment of your time and energy, you need more support in the beginning. Then, as you feel more confident about your new lifestyle, only occasional assistance will be necessary to maintain your healthier habits and keep the momentum going.

In this chapter, you'll learn how to attach your own training wheels—your support system—to your diabetes and weight management plan. You'll start by evaluating your current support network. Then you'll identify ways you can support yourself, learn how to choose at least one health partner to strengthen your program, and develop the skills necessary to ask for assistance from others.

Building Support

They say the depth of a foundation determines how high a building will be. This saying also applies to your support system. To succeed, you need to spend time laying your foundation (self-care) and strengthening it with family, friends, coworkers, and your health care team. Changes in lifestyle take into account not only who you are as a person but also the environment in which you live. As a result, you need to gather strength from within (internal support) and create the proper environment (external support) to prosper. The stronger your network, the more successful you'll be.

Internal support means taking care of yourself. Self-care is the core component of your circle. But what is self-care? It's taking a positive, proactive approach to care for your physical and mental health. Each day, you make a conscious choice to put your health needs first because you believe you deserve it. Belief in yourself gives you the strength to move forward in reaching your health goals.

But it's going to take more than just belief in yourself. You need to create a supportive environment, because other people in your surroundings, such as family and friends, can be either your best supporters or your worst enemies. As you start to make changes in your eating and exercise habits, your friends and family are bound to be impacted by them. For example, if you have always made the same 10 recipes and suddenly add new, healthier ones to your repertoire, you start to disturb the day-to-day routine. Your family may accept the change or rebel by trying to undermine your efforts. Friends can react in a similar manner. For example, you might have a friend you go to a movie with every Friday. Traditionally, you order popcorn, a box of your favorite candy, and a soda. Now that you're trying to lose weight, you make a conscious decision to skip the snacks. Your friend can either support you by agreeing to skip the treats (or buy his or her own and eat them quietly) or tempt you by frequently offering you some.

These are just a few examples of how other people in your external support circle—family, friends, and coworkers—can help or hinder your success. There are other groups or individuals who can join your circle to provide ongoing support for your efforts (See the Circle of Support). Your health care team is a great example. They understand the changes you're going through and can offer ideas on where to seek additional support when you need help sticking with your goals. An aerobics class may be just the solution to keep you on track with your exercise routine, or a visit with another patient who has taken the path you're embarking on might inspire you. Let them support and guide you as you continue on your journey.

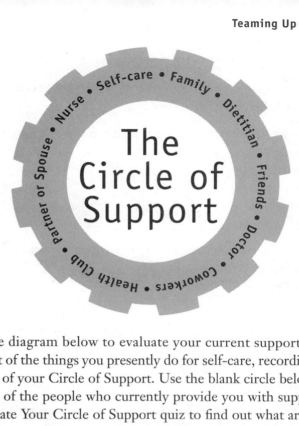

Use the diagram below to evaluate your current support structure. Make a list of the things you presently do for self-care, recording them in the center of your Circle of Support. Use the blank circle below to write the names of the people who currently provide you with support. Then take the Rate Your Circle of Support quiz to find out what areas of your foundation are weak, if any, so that you can improve your circle of support.

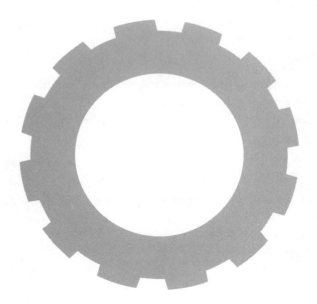

Rate Your Circle of Support

For each item, circle the one response that best describes your current support network. Then total the scores.

When you have a health-related problem, do you discuss it with other people? How many?

_____ none (0)

_____ one or two (3)

_____ two or three (4)

_____ four or more (5)

Do you ask for help with grocery shopping, cooking, yard work, car maintenance, and other household chores?

_____ no (0)

_____ yes (3)

Do you have a partner, spouse, friend, or family member who is also interested in health?

_____ no (0)

_____ yes (10)

Do close family members or friends exercise with you or encourage you to maintain health habits? How often?

_____ rarely (0)

_____ about once a month (1)

_____ several times a month (4)

_____ once a week or more (8)

Do you talk with family members or friends about your diabetes or weight management program? How many?

_____ none (0)

_____ one or two (6)

_____ three to five (8)

_____ six or more (10)

Do you believe you will succeed in managing your diabetes and your weight?

_____ no (0)

_____ yes (10)

Now evaluate your score. If your score is:

Less than 15: Your circle probably doesn't offer much help. Use the tips in the upcoming pages to enlist the support of family and friends as you continue your efforts in weight and diabetes management.

15 to 29: Your network probably provides enough support for day-to-day living, but not enough during periods of high stress and change. You need others most when you're feeling pressured and pulled in too many directions. Don't be afraid to ask for assistance from others during these times. Positive encouragement and a healthy environment make life easier all the time.

30 or more: The foundation of your support system is strong, and your network of family, friends, and coworkers will help you maintain your well-being and health habits even during periods of high stress and change.

If your score puts you in either of the first two groups, there are steps you can take to build a stronger circle. The following are several key strategies that will help you create a successful support network.

Strategy 1: Practice Self-Care

Taking care of yourself is often a difficult task with today's fast-paced lifestyles. It's too easy to push your own health and well-being aside and give freely to others. Yet self-care does begin with you. A positive and supportive environment really is essential for success.

One of the best self-care practices is believing in yourself. Self-efficacy is the perception that you can achieve your goal, whether it's sticking with an exercise routine, recording your blood glucose levels, or taking a 15-minute relaxation break each day. Henry Ford once said, "Whether you think you can or you can't—you are right." You're much more likely to rise to any challenge or change and reach your goal if you have a strong belief in your ability to do so. Several factors that can contribute to your self-efficacy are past attempts and successes at reaching your goal, seeing others with similar goals achieve them, and encouragement from others in your support circle. Affirmations (positive statements you tell yourself that describe who you are and what you want to become) can also help. Write a list of supportive statements and refer to it regularly throughout the day. Review the example list to get some ideas before making your own personal list.

Affirmations

I am filled with self-confidence.

I take good care of myself because I'm worth it.

Mistakes are unavoidable and human. I can accept my being human.

I am becoming better and better at my new health habits.

I am important to my friends, family, and most of all to myself.

I will succeed in achieving my diabetes and weight management goals.

My personal affirmations are...

_____

_____

_____

_____

_____

Additionally, self-care extends beyond your belief in yourself. To continue to succeed, you need to learn how to assert yourself with others to prevent them from sabotaging your ongoing efforts. Creating a supportive environment that guarantees success is up to you. If coworkers frequently bring goodies to work, or keep candy dishes out on their desks, ask them to respect your health goals by keeping them out of sight. If friends and family frequently talk about the food choices you make or the exercise session you missed, request that they discuss your habits positively, focusing on the progress you've made thus far.

You may be familiar with the saying "you are what you eat," and a similar saying applies to your environment: "You are as positive and as successful as the people and the environment in which you live." Make your choices wisely.

Strategy 2: Choose a Supportive Partner

Other people have an influential role in how well you manage your weight and diabetes. When you're experiencing high levels of stress or change, a partner can support you with encouraging words—words that remind you how wonderful you are and that you're making progress. Your partner can empathize with you. Maintaining a healthy lifestyle can be challenging, and he or she struggles, too. A partner listens and reminds you that it will get easier. If you need help sticking to your exercise program, he or she is willing to get your momentum moving forward again by offering to exercise with you. Remember, a partner doesn't have to limit support to difficult times; a partner supports you day-in-and-day-out.

Keep in mind, however, that choosing a partner to assist you in maintaining health habits doesn't guarantee he or she will provide the kind of support you need. Sometimes people want to help you, but they don't know how. Or, although it's not intentional, they say they'll encourage you, but instead they criticize you or act as if they are policing your every move.

When you select a support person—whether it's a spouse, significant other, or friend—you want to feel comfortable sharing your diabetes and weight management goals. Here are some attributes of supportive people you should look for to select a companion who will be truly supportive:

Easy to talk to about health goals or setbacks

Expresses concern about his or her own health

Understands the difficulties of managing weight or diabetes

Displays a genuine interest in helping you

Thinks positively

Provides encouragement on a regular basis

Offers support, whether it's listening or helping with household chores

If you have someone in your life who has most or all of these attributes, it's likely you've found an ideal support person. If you can't think of anyone who fits the description, try to seek out someone who has these characteristics. Keep in mind that no one person can provide you with all the support you need. It takes many people to build your circle.

Continue enhancing your circle by seeking additional support from people who have similar goals or issues. Being around others who are experiencing the same issues as you is a validating experience. It's nice to know you're not alone. If you don't like groups, see a dietitian, exercise physiologist, or therapist one-on-one for additional help. If you like groups, there are lots of options. You can attend a commercial program such as TOPS (Taking Off Pounds Sensibly) or Weight Watchers. If you want to share your experiences in diabetes management with others, contact your hospital, clinic, or the local affiliate of the American Diabetes Association to get involved in a support group. For exercise, you can join a local health club, mall walking club, or community education class. The options are endless; what you choose depends on what you identify your needs to be.

Strategy 3: Teach Others How to Support You

As mentioned earlier, choosing a partner or sharing your goals with others doesn't guarantee you'll get the kind of support you need. Sometimes people mean well, but they hurt or hinder rather than help your efforts. For instance, Janie has been trying diligently to lower her fat intake. She's been purposefully eating fewer sweets and high-fat snacks such as chips. Although Janie has been making progress, the habits of her husband, John, have not made her efforts easy. Knowing full well that she has difficulty saying no to temptations, he frequently eats potato chips in front of her when they watch TV together. He also brings home sweet rolls and cookies from the local bakery on a regular basis. Although John indicates that he's supportive of Janie's efforts, his behaviors are sabotaging her goals.

Another case in point is Bert. Every Sunday afternoon his family gets together for dinner. Sounds nonthreatening enough, right? Yet Bert dreads these weekly gatherings. From the moment the meal begins, his wife and kids watch every mouthful he eats. They make comments such as "you shouldn't eat that, it has sugar and you're a diabetic." "No wonder you don't lose weight, look at how much you eat." Although Bert's family says they are only trying to help, their comments only cause him more anguish and frustration.

You may be able to relate to these examples. These situations are difficult because it's often hard to tell family and friends how you really feel. You don't want them to get upset or angry with you. However, if you're

---

What if my success in losing weight makes my family or friends feel jealous and uncomfortable?

NO QUESTION IS SILLY

This is not an uncommon reaction. As you take control of your health, others may realize they need to do the same, especially if they're overweight, too. But they may not be ready for it and act as though they don't want things to change. They could also feel that the new, thinner you is going to leave them or like them less. Just as you need reinforcement from them about your progress and the positive changes you've made, others need encouragement and support from you. Praise them for their support and remind them how important they are to your success. If they express interest in making changes in their lifestyle habits, offer to share what you've learned and likewise be a positive, reinforcing voice in their lives.

going to continue to be successful in maintaining your health habits, you need to learn how to respond appropriately in these situations to create a positive environment. The key is practicing assertive responses. An easy way to remember the steps involved in responding assertively is to use the DESC model. The components of the model are

Describe the behavior that is bothersome to you.

Effect it is having on you, both behaviorally and emotionally.

Specify what you would like changed.

Consequences of this change for you. How will you feel if the person does what you request?

To understand this model better, it might be helpful to review the first example with Janie. How could Janie assertively tell John that his habits make it difficult for her to stick with her fat gram goal? Using the DESC model, here is how she could respond to the situation:

Describe: "John, you frequently bring home many high-fat snacks and sweets."

Effect: "I'm feeling frustrated by the temptation they present and how you always eat them in front of me. I don't feel you're supportive of my effort to maintain my low-fat meal plan."

Specify: "I'd appreciate it if you'd stop buying high-fat sweets and snacks, bringing them home, and eating them in front of me."

Consequences: "If you'd stop buying them or eat them when I'm not around, I'd feel as if you were more supportive of my efforts to lose weight, which is extremely important to my health. I really value your encouragement."

How do you feel about Janie's response to John's behavior? Responding in this manner may feel uncomfortable at first, but as with anything, practice makes it easier and easier. To get practice using the DESC model, use the Take Control Work Sheet on page 100. As you complete the work sheet, consider the following tips that will help you become more assertive in getting the support you need:

Acknowledge others when they give you support. Tell them how much you appreciate them and their help. They'll be more apt to continue with their positive behaviors, and so will you. It's a win-win situation for both of you.

Express yourself by using words that describe your feelings instead of using neutral terms. For example, say, "I like this salad" or "I don't want any dessert, I'm not hungry" rather than "This salad is good" or " Just give me a little piece because I'm not very hungry right now." You can also use words like "I think" or "I feel" if it's fitting.

Learn to be comfortable talking about yourself. It's okay to share your health achievements with family and friends.

Make eye contact. Try to look people directly in the eye when talking to them.

State disagreements. Use words such as "I have a different outlook on that matter, all foods can be eaten in small quantities."

Be persistent. Don't give up easily if you really believe in something.

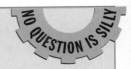

My doctor accuses me of not trying hard enough to lose weight. How can I make my doctor see that I am making positive health changes?

Your doctor is an integral member of your support team. To show your progress, you may want to bring in your food records or discuss your goals and weekly action plans. Learn to respond to any negativity in an assertive manner—no different than with anyone else. Refer back to the DESC model. Your conversation may go something like this:

Describe: "Dr. Smith, you've asked me several times if I'm really sticking to my diabetes and weight management goals."

Effect: "I'm feeling perplexed about your repeated questioning. You don't seem to believe me when I tell you I'm really trying."

Specify: "I'd sincerely appreciate it if you'd stop telling me that I'm not trying."

Consequences: "If you'd stop telling me I'm not trying and instead acknowledge the progress I've made thus far, I'd really feel as if you were supporting my efforts to improve my health. Your support is very important to me."

In this chapter, you've learned how to strengthen your self-care, which is the core of your circle. You've also identified ways to foster additional support from others. How you choose to continue building and maintaining health habits is your decision. For some individuals, inner strength keeps their momentum going, and for others it's the encouragement of other people. Ultimately the responsibility of managing your diabetes and weight is up to you. So devise a plan that helps you get what you need.

Take Control Work Sheet

The following situation (at work, home, other) makes it difficult for me to maintain healthy habits important to my weight and diabetes management:

_____

_____

_____

_____

Using the DESC model, I can respond to these situations as follows:

Describe: _____

_____

Effect: _____

_____

Specify: _____

_____

Consequences: _____

_____

Assertive statements I can use to ask my partner, family, friends, or co-workers for support:

_____

_____

_____

_____

_____

_____

_____

_____

keeping pace with exercise

"I can't do it" never yet accomplished anything; "I will try" has performed wonders.
George P. Burnham

AN ACTION PLAN

Once you've started being active on a day-to-day basis, it's important to begin adding the other components of your all-star program—aerobic, stretching, and strengthening exercises—to improve your weight loss and diabetes management.

In this chapter you'll learn how much, how often, how hard, and when to do aerobic exercise, strength conditioning, and stretching to manage your diabetes control and your weight and to maximize your health. You'll also learn how to identify the personal barriers you may have to exercise and develop strategies to get moving and stay motivated.

Aerobic Exercise—Your Prescription

Exercise—like medications—can have a significant impact on your health. Aerobic exercise is important to your weight management program because it promotes fat loss. Like other components of your all-star activity program, aerobic exercise can result in decreased blood glucose levels, lower weight, increased "good" cholesterol levels, and lower blood pressure—all health benefits people also receive from medication. So treat aerobic exercise like the pills your doctor prescribes. Here's how:

Be Consistent. Exercising regularly is what really counts. Plan each day to get your 30-minute dose of lifestyle activity (as discussed in chapter 4). Every week, schedule aerobic exercises such as biking, walking, or swimming on your calendar. Before starting, remember to check with your health care provider about any exercise restrictions. Gradually increase your exercise dosage to the recommended amount—based on frequency, intensity, and time.

Frequency refers to how often you exercise. To lose weight and manage your diabetes, aim for three to five sessions of aerobic exercise each week.

Intensity refers to how hard you exercise. You can measure this by determining your target heart rate or using the Exercise Intensity Meter (see below). Exercise should feel somewhat hard—but not strenuous—to maximize the benefit to your heart. You are exercising too hard if you can't carry on a normal conversation with a friend.

Time refers to how long you exercise. Your diabetes and weight management plan recommends exercising between 20 and 60 minutes per session. How long you decide to exercise depends on your current activity level. If you're a beginner, start out by exercising 5 to 10 minutes per session. If you've been doing some activity, you may want to aim for 20 minutes. Gradually increase the number of minutes you exercise to the maximum recommended amount.

Take as Directed. Every time you exercise, you should start with a warm-up, then stretch your muscles before participating in an aerobic activity. Don't forget to cool down and finish your session by stretching again. Each component is necessary not only to achieve your health and fitness goals but to prevent injury as well. Page 103 shows a chart listing each component of an aerobic exercise session, why it's important, and the recommended time per session for each.

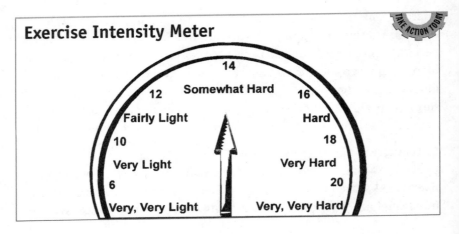

Monitor Your Exercise Dosage. When you take any type of medication, you don't want to take too much or too little. The same is true for exercise. If your diabetes has been in good control, exercise will lower your blood glucose level. So, remember to check it before and after an exercise session to determine if you need some food to counteract a low blood glucose reading. Ask your health care provider when the best time for you to exercise is and whether he or she recommends food before, during, or after your session based on your prescribed medication. If you exercise for more than an hour at a time, check blood glucose levels during the exercise session.

Take With Food. Occasionally some medications require you take them with food or just after a meal. For most people with Type II diabetes, the preferred time to exercise to prevent low blood glucose levels is about 1 to 2 hours after meals—when your blood glucose levels are at their highest—or in the morning if your blood glucose levels tend to be high.

If you take insulin, you will most likely need to take food before exercise. (Ask your health care provider for more detailed instructions on when and what to eat.) If you take medication for your diabetes, or take nothing at all, it's very likely you won't need to take additional food. But to be safe, follow these guidelines:

Eat a snack, such as a serving of fruit, bread, or milk from the Food Guide Pyramid, when your blood glucose level is less than 100 mg./dl. before periods of exercise lasting less than an hour.

Skip the snack when your blood glucose level is between 100 and 150 mg./dl.

Exercise Session: Start to Finish

ACTIVITY	WHY DO IT?	FOR HOW LONG?
Warm-up	Gets the body ready for exercise	3 to 5 minutes
Stretching	Prepares the muscles for exercise	3 to 5 minutes
Aerobic activity	Improves how your heart and lungs work and burns calories to promote weight loss or weight maintenance	20 to 60 minutes
Cooldown	Gradually slows down your heart rate and decreases your blood pressure after aerobic activity	3 to 5 minutes
Stretching	Reduces muscle soreness	3 to 5 minutes

Check with your physician if you have blood glucose levels above 250 mg./dl. You may be advised not to exercise when your blood glucose is this high.

Know the side effects. Because exercise can decrease your blood glucose levels, it's important that you be aware of how you're feeling. Typically you'll feel symptoms (dizziness, shaking, sweating) of hypoglycemia when your blood glucose drops below 70 mg./dl. Carry some fast-acting sugar (glucose tabs, fruit, etc.) with you just in case your blood glucose levels get low. Drink about 1/2 cup of water for every 15 minutes of exercise to maintain your hydration.

Understand the precautions. If you have neuropathy, retinopathy, high blood pressure, nephropathy, or a heart condition, or if your blood glucose levels are poorly controlled (typically higher than 250 mg./dl.), check with your health care team for specific activity guidelines before beginning to exercise.

Measuring Your Intensity

Once you start exercising, you may wonder whether you're exercising hard enough. As mentioned earlier, part of your exercise prescription is determining how hard you're working each time you do aerobic exercise. There are two ways to measure the intensity of your workout: target heart rate and perceived exertion.

The first way to measure your exercise intensity (how hard you're working) is by checking your heart rate. Your heart rate, measured in beats per minute, usually relates closely to the amount of work your body is doing when you exercise. To measure your heart rate, count the number of times your heart beats in one minute. You can do this by using your finger (but not your thumb) to take your pulse at your wrist near the joint of the thumb and wrist. If you can't find your pulse on your wrist, measure it at your neck next to your Adam's apple.

Check your pulse while exercising or immediately upon stopping. Count the beats for 10 seconds and then check the Target Heart Rate Chart (page 105) to see where you should be at for your age. If you've been sedentary up until now, your heart rate should be in the 50 to 60 percent training zone. Aim for 60 to 70 percent if you've been exercising some but not regularly. The ultimate goal, once you're consistent with your exercise

Target Heart Rate Chart

BEATS PER 10 SECONDS

AGE	50%	60%	70%	85%
20	17	20	23	28
25	16	20	23	28
30	16	19	22	27
35	15	19	22	26
40	15	18	21	26
45	15	18	20	25
50	14	17	20	24
55	14	17	19	23
60	13	16	19	23
65	13	16	18	22
70	13	15	18	21
75	12	15	17	21
80	12	14	16	20

program, is to keep your heart rate between 70 and 85 percent of your maximum heart rate. Target heart rate is calculated by subtracting your age from 220 and multiplying the result by the percentage of your maximum heart rate you want to achieve (60 to 85 percent).

Example: 40-year-old wants to exercise at 70 percent. $220 - 40 = 180$
$180 \times 0.70 = 126$
$126 \div 6 = 21$ (target heart rate for a 10-second count)

There are some exceptions to using this formula. If you have neuropathy, for example, or take medications for high blood pressure that may affect your heart rate response to exercise, you may need to listen to your body signals to determine how hard you're working.

To use body signals to rate how hard you're working, use the Exercise Intensity Meter (also called *perceived exertion*). This meter (page 102) relates to your target heart rate but focuses on how you're feeling during exercise.

Think of the Exercise Intensity Meter as being similar to your car's speedometer. When you drive your car on the highway, you don't drive at the fastest speed your car can go. You usually aim for 50 to 65 MPH—the speed at which it's most fuel efficient (and, of course, within the speed limit). Your body works the same way. To gain the most benefits for your heart, you want your meter to register at 11 to 15. If you've been fairly sedentary, start with a speed in the 11 to 13 range. If you're active already, aim for 13 to 15. You should try not to start above 15 because you may tire easily, put yourself at risk of injury, or increase your potential for hypoglycemia if you take insulin or another medication for your diabetes.

As you're exercising, ask yourself: "How hard am I exercising?" You want your exercise effort to feel "somewhat hard." If you can't carry on a normal conversation while exercising, you've exceeded your speed limit. Slow down.

Strengthen Your Program

Aerobic exercise is important, but don't forget that strengthening exercises are also a part of your all-star activity program. Strengthening exercises help you build and preserve muscle strength. Although you may envision muscle-bound weight lifters when you think of strength conditioning, you don't have to lift massive amounts of weight to get benefits. These exercises help you tone and shape your body as well as lose weight. The more muscle you have, the more calories you'll burn. Adding 1 pound of muscle burns 30 to 50 extra calories per day.

Strength conditioning is especially important as you get older because muscle is your body's primary calorie burner. As you age, you gradually lose muscle mass (about 3 to 6 percent every 10 years, beginning at age 30), which means your metabolism will slow down, causing you to burn fewer calories. You can minimize loss of muscle mass by making strengthening exercises a part of your activity plan.

Strengthening exercises include calisthenics such as sit-ups and push-ups or weight training—working your muscles against moderate resistance. The resistance can be provided by free weights (dumbbells or

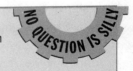

If I wear extra clothing during exercise so that I sweat more, or sit in the sauna after a workout at the health club, will I lose more weight?

Sorry—neither will help you lose weight. Although you may initially see a decrease in weight due to loss of body fluids such as water, when you replenish the fluids your body has lost, your weight will return to its pre-exercise level. Bear in mind that neither of these practices is safe. They make your heart beat faster and affect your body's heat regulation system.

barbells), resistance or rubber bands, weight machines at the health club, or household items such as shampoo bottles or cans of soup. Before beginning these exercises, remember to warm up for 3 to 5 minutes, then do stretching exercises. When you're done, remember to cool down and stretch, too. You may want to meet with an exercise specialist at your health club or schedule an appointment with an exercise physiologist that your health care provider recommends to set up a specific program. These professionals can help you learn how to lift properly and tell you the type and amount of weight to use. Do these exercises every other day. Muscles need 48 hours of rest between sessions. Caution: if you have retinopathy, avoid weight lifting and ask your health care provider for strengthening exercises that are safe for you.

Be Flexible

Stretching is another essential, and often forgotten, component of your all-star activity program. Stretching is important because it keeps your body flexible and joints mobile, reducing your risk of injury. Although stretching exercises are an important part of your aerobic and strength-conditioning workout, it's recommended you do some every day to stay limber and reduce muscle tension.

When you stretch, try to work all the muscles in your body, such as your arms, back, neck, stomach, hips, and legs. To prevent injury, warm up by walking before stretching. Avoid bouncing when you're doing a stretch. Stretch only until comfortable, not painful. Hold each stretch for at least 10 seconds. Remember that you don't need to hold your breath. Stretching is important both before and after exercise because it keeps muscles from tightening up.

Break the Barriers

Although knowing the recommendations for exercise is important, following them can be difficult. You may be motivated to start leading an active lifestyle, but unless you do a little planning and develop a positive "I can do it" attitude, it's tough to make exercise a permanent habit. As you learned in chapter 6, you need to set realistic goals and determine action steps that spell success. Exercise doesn't just happen. You need time, energy, and motivation to keep exercise at the top of your priority list.

If you haven't started adding activity or exercise to your health routine, and aren't sure why, review the Barriers to Exercise Checklist and then read on to determine which strategies can help you start or maintain a physically active lifestyle.

Barriers to Exercise Checklist

The following barriers commonly prevent people from leading active lifestyles. Check all the statements that apply to you:

Fear of Injury

_____ I'm too old to exercise, I might get injured.

_____ I don't know how to exercise properly and could get hurt.

_____ I have an old high school injury that might flare up.

_____ Before I start, I need to check with my doctor, and I can't get an appointment until next month.

_____ I feel stiff when I start exercising, so I don't do it.

Lack of Energy

_____ I'm too tired to exercise when I get done with work.

I'm frequently out of town for work. Any suggestions on how to get activity on the road?

NO QUESTION IS SILLY

You can start by calling hotels in advance and choosing only those that offer fitness facilities. Make sure to pack appropriate workout clothing, depending on whether indoor exercise facilities are available and what the weather conditions are at your destination. If your travel involves flying, try walking around the airport instead of sitting while you wait. Once you arrive at your destination, make an effort to walk to restaurants or meetings as much as possible. Check to see if there are any exercise programs on TV. You may even want to pack a jump rope or an elastic band and try stretching before bed. All of these activities will help you stick with your all-star activity program.

_____ When I exercise at night, I'm too awake to sleep.

_____ I can't get up any earlier in the morning.

Lack of Resources

_____ There are no walking paths or trails near my home.

_____ It's too expensive to buy good exercise shoes.

_____ I can't afford to join a health club or buy equipment to use at home.

_____ I don't have a VCR at home for exercise videos.

Lack of Skill

_____ When I was younger, I wasn't good at sports.

_____ It's hard to learn new skills at my age.

_____ I don't feel comfortable going to the health club because I'm not as slender or as coordinated as other people there.

Lack of Time

_____ I'm just too busy to exercise.

_____ If I try to squeeze exercise in to my hectic schedule, I'll never have time for my family.

_____ It takes too much time to drive to a health club or a shopping mall.

Lack of Motivation

_____ I'm seriously thinking about exercise, but I just can't seem to get started.

_____ I have a different reason each day for why I don't exercise.

_____ I hate exercising—it's not fun.

_____ I never stick with it, so why bother.

Now it's time to review your assessment. Did you check all the statements under a specific barrier? If so, that may be the one area you want to focus on first. If you checked quite a few statements in many different areas, develop strategies such as the following for one barrier at a time and use them as action steps in the weeks ahead.

Listed on the following pages are examples of different barriers and some potential action steps for your use in the upcoming weeks. Depending on your personal situation, there may be many more action steps or strategies you could try. Use the blank spaces to add your own ideas.

Fear of Injury

Check with your health care provider if you have physical limitations or special conditions (for example, retinopathy or neuropathy) that may limit the types of activity in which you choose to participate.

Start with something simple, familiar, and fun, such as walking.

Work with an exercise physiologist or certified personal trainer to develop a plan that's comfortable to you.

Exercise properly. Remember to warm up and stretch before exercising and cool down and stretch again when you're done. You can avoid injury by building up your exercise level gradually.

Take an exercise class.

Other _____

_____

_____

Lack of Energy

Exercise when you feel the most energetic.

Set realistic expectations. Sneak in some exercise regularly and evaluate how you feel. Most people find that once they start exercising, they have more energy.

Other _____

_____

_____

Lack of Resources

Try activities that aren't expensive such as walking in your neighborhood or at the mall, hiking at a nearby park, or doing an exercise video at home.

Evaluate community education classes or activities available at work. They may be offered at low or no cost.

Rent or lease equipment.

Shop for used exercise equipment in the newspaper or secondhand stores.

Check out your local YMCA. They often offer scholarships.

Other _____

_____

_____

Lack of Skill

Take a class to learn a new activity or sport.

Be assertive and ask friends to teach you a sport they're good at.

Decide to do activities that don't require a lot of skill, such as walking or hiking.

Other _____

_____

_____

Does exercise really turn my fat into muscle?

NO QUESTION IS SILLY

Fat can't turn to muscle, and muscle can't turn to fat. When you exercise, however, you can decrease your body fat and increase your muscle mass. To build and maintain your muscle tissue, you need to incorporate strengthening exercises such as lifting free weights, doing sit-ups and pull-ups, and using resistance or rubber bands. The more muscle you have, the more calories your body will burn. If your goal is to lose fat and tone muscles, you need to do aerobic exercises such as biking, jogging, or stair climbing. Both strengthening and aerobic exercises are important components of your all-star activity program.

Lack of Time

Schedule exercise into your daily routine—no different than work or dinner parties.

Go for a walk at lunch break or just after work.

Delegate some household tasks such as cooking or picking up the dry cleaning so that you have more time to exercise.

Plan to get at least two exercise sessions on the weekend when your days are less structured.

Other _____

_____

_____

Lack of Motivation

Find an exercise partner—a partner makes you more accountable and motivates you.

Tell everyone at work when you're going to exercise. It will increase your motivation to do it.

Set out your exercise clothes in the morning so that when you get home, you'll be encouraged to work out.

Visualize yourself exercising. If you can see yourself doing it, you will do it!

Other _____

_____

I do 50 sit-ups every night, but I still can't lose inches around my waist. Why?

NO QUESTION IS SILLY

What you're experiencing is common. Many people think that spot reducing can remove fat from around their middle, but this method actually doesn't work. Doing sit-ups won't remove the fat from your middle or burn very many calories. This doesn't mean, however, that you shouldn't do sit-ups. Because they tone your stomach and strengthen your abdominal muscles, sit-ups are an important part of back care. You need to do aerobic exercise to burn body fat.

Writing Your Exercise Prescription

Now it's time to develop an action plan. The first step is determining what types of activities you're already doing. Review the All-Star Activity Logs you've been keeping since chapter 4. Have you made more attempts to increase activity in your daily routine? Were you already doing some aerobic exercise? What activities are you missing from your all-star activity program?

Next, on a sheet of paper, list all the activities you enjoy—whether they're lifestyle, leisure, aerobic, strengthening, or stretching exercises. Once you've completed your list, identify the missing points of your activity star. If you're already getting 30 minutes of lifestyle activity each day, but no aerobic exercise, this may be where you want to start.

After you've decided where you'd like to begin, start including weekly action steps targeted at exercise. Record them on the Take Action, Make It Happen work sheets from chapter 6 or continue to use the All-Star Activity Log (page 114) to track the changes you're making in your activity habits. When you do aerobic exercise, record your heart rate or exercise intensity as another way to measure progress. Keep in mind that building up endurance with each new activity you do takes time.

As you continue moving forward, periodically assess how you're doing and where you're going with your all-star activity program. Review successes as well as setbacks and gradually increase your exercise and activity to the recommended amounts. Try not to put yourself down if you miss a day or don't achieve your weekly action steps. Just remind yourself "I can do it" and get back to your routine the next day. Success sometimes comes by repeatedly taking two steps forward and one step back.

All-Star Activity Log

ACTIVITY	MINUTES	TOTAL	HEART RATE OR EXERCISE INTENSITY
stretching	10		
aerobics class	30		15
walking at work	10	50 min.	

Monday

Tuesday

Wednesday

Thursday

Friday

Saturday

Sunday

To record additional days, photocopy this page.

nutrition extras

**It's what you learn after
you know it all that counts.**
Anonymous

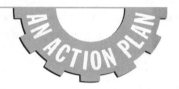

When you were first diagnosed with diabetes, you probably thought you just needed to worry about sugar—specifically, eating as little sugar as possible. But now you know there's more to it. Living with diabetes involves many nutrition factors—having regularly planned meals and snacks, getting consistent amounts of carbohydrate at the same meal each day, and tracking calories—to name a few. You can prioritize healthy eating habits into three levels of importance:

Level 1—The Healthy Basics. You need food for the energy and 40-plus nutrients it provides to keep your body running properly day-to-day.

Level 2—The Reduction Factor. Efforts are made to eat less of "negative" nutrients such as fat and sodium because they contribute to chronic diseases such as cancer and heart disease.

Level 3—The Fountain of Health. More and more, you notice products on the grocery store shelves with nutrients intentionally added to them to give a health benefit. Examples include orange juice with added calcium, bread with folic acid, and peanut butter with eight minerals and vitamins.

What you've read so far has given you good coverage of level 1. You know the basics of a healthy eating plan for persons with diabetes. Because you have concerns about weight management, you're working on level 2 by cutting back on calories and fat. As you move through this chapter you'll learn even more about nutrition factors in levels 2 and 3 and will be well on your way to becoming a nutrition expert, personalizing even more your eating plan for weight and diabetes management. To expand your nutrition horizons, the topics of dietary fat, sodium, fiber, alcohol, and vitamins and minerals are covered in this chapter.

Fat Is Where It's At

You've heard it from your health care provider and friends who also have diabetes, and you've read it in pamphlets—cardiovascular disease is the number one killer of persons with diabetes. But this doesn't mean it has to happen to you. Several of the factors that increase the risk of heart disease are controllable.

The amount and type of fat you eat affect your blood cholesterol levels—one of the controllable risk factors for heart disease. The goal is to lower your fat intake to less than 30 percent of your total calories. This not only helps with weight control but also can lower blood cholesterol levels. The type of fat you eat makes an even bigger difference. A description of the three types of fat and how each affects your blood cholesterol follows.

Saturated fat is the real culprit in raising blood cholesterol levels. All animal products—meats, poultry, cheese, and milk—have some saturated fat. Other sources include solid fats such as lard, butter, and margarine, and tropical oils such as palm and palm kernel oil. To lower blood cholesterol levels, the initial goal is to limit saturated fat to no more than 10 percent of your calories. Once you're comfortable at this level, dropping it to 7 percent of calories may result in even greater reductions in your blood cholesterol levels.

You may wonder whether it is better to count total fat grams or saturated fat grams. For lowering blood cholesterol, saturated fat is the most important to limit. But because you're also concerned about weight control, you want to focus on cutting back on total fat as well. If you're limiting the high-fat foods you eat, you may already be within the recommended guidelines for saturated fat. Track saturated fat for a few days by reading food labels (see chapter 11) on products you use. If you're below 7 percent of calories from saturated fat, you don't need to track saturated fat grams separately from total fat grams.

Because margarine and butter both have saturated fat, there is continuing debate about which you should use. The main ingredient in margarine is a liquid oil, which is turned to a solid spread through hydrogenation. As a part of this process, the liquid oil becomes more saturated. However, because it has less saturated fat, margarine is still a better choice than butter. Choose tub margarines, those called "reduced fat," and those with water listed as the first ingredient for the lowest saturated-fat content. Keep in mind the overall goal—to use less of all fats, including margarine and butter.

Polyunsaturated fat is found in vegetable oils, specifically corn, soybean, sunflower, safflower, and cottonseed oils. They're all liquid at room temperature. When used to replace saturated fats in your meals and snacks, polyunsaturated fats can lower blood cholesterol levels. This substitution not only can help lower total blood cholesterol levels but also lowers LDL-cholesterol, the so-called bad cholesterol. The goal is for one-third of your fat calories to come from polyunsaturated fat.

Monounsaturated fats come from vegetable sources. Canola, olive, and peanut oils are high in monounsaturated fats. As with using polyunsaturates, using monounsaturated fats instead of saturated fats will help lower total and LDL-cholesterol levels. Up to 15 percent of your calories can come from monounsaturated fat. People native to Mediterranean countries tend to have lower cholesterol levels than are found in the United States. One reason may be that they eat a higher percent of olive oil than polyunsaturated or saturated fats, a part of the so-called Mediterranean diet.

These are the only kinds of fat found in foods. Another term often confused with fat is *dietary cholesterol*. Cholesterol is like a cousin to fat but is different in many ways. It doesn't have any calories and is found only in animal products (meats, milk, eggs, cheese, etc.). Some people think that cholesterol is a fat, however, because of its role in heart disease.

Your body gets cholesterol in two ways—from the food you eat (dietary cholesterol) and from production by your liver. Your liver uses saturated fat to make cholesterol. Even if you don't eat any cholesterol, your body still makes it. Ten years ago, medical professionals thought eating too much cholesterol was causing heart disease. But today they know saturated fat plays a much larger role. Dietary cholesterol should, however, still be limited to less than 300 milligrams per day.

Although cutting back on total fat is probably routine for you by now, you might not have given much thought to limiting saturated fat. The following Take Action Today tips can help you lower your saturated fat intake and your risk of heart disease. Consider using these tips in the months ahead as weekly action steps. Refer to appendixes B and C for hints to lower fat while grocery shopping and when cooking your favorite recipes.

Take Action Today

While at the grocery store, look at the saturated-fat content of foods you usually buy. Consider trying similar products with a lower saturated-fat number on the label.

When browning ground meats for use in casseroles, spaghetti, or tacos, drain the oil and rinse the meat under hot water.

Use liquid oils instead of solid fats whenever possible. In quick bread and muffin recipes, use 7/8 cup liquid oil for every cup of butter or margarine. Or try applesauce, prune baby food, or fat-free yogurt as a substitute for half or all the fat in these recipes.

Use margarines with liquid oil or water listed as the first ingredient. Try using reduced-fat, reduced-calorie, or diet margarines.

Limit portion sizes of meats to a daily maximum of 6 ounces.

If you make homemade soups or stews, refrigerate them overnight to let the fat harden on top. Skim it off, reheat, and serve.

Choose meatless meals two to three times a week.

Use skim milk instead of cream in coffee. Order your lattes and caffe au lait "skinny, no whip" (made with skim milk and served without whipped cream).

Seasoning for Health

Whereas eating too much saturated fat increases blood cholesterol levels, thus increasing your risk of heart disease, sodium affects blood pressure—another of the controllable risk factors for heart disease. Not everyone is sensitive to sodium, but for those who are, limiting sodium in foods they eat can lower their blood pressure and possibly even prevent the need for medication.

If you already have high blood pressure, see if reducing the sodium you eat helps. If you don't have high blood pressure, there is no test you can take to tell if you are sodium sensitive—that having too much sodium will contribute to high blood pressure. So you may want to limit the amount of sodium you eat as a precautionary measure.

But how low do you go? Most health organizations recommend 2,400 milligrams of sodium a day. Because this is half the sodium that most people currently eat, this guideline may seem too restrictive. Just remember, any changes you make to lower sodium in the foods you eat can be beneficial.

Sodium comes from three different sources: it occurs naturally in foods such as celery and in processed foods such as canned vegetables, soups, and frozen entrées, and it is added during cooking or at the table in the form of salt. One teaspoon of salt contains close to the amount of sodium you should have for the entire day. When considering where to cut back on sodium, think about your own habits. Do you salt most of your foods? How often do you use canned vegetables? Do you read food labels for sodium as well as for fat? Using these questions to assess your own habits will give you ideas on where to make changes.

For most people, the toughest battle in limiting sodium is in convenience foods. Few people have time to cook from scratch anymore. Convenience is a reality in today's fast-paced world. So finding a variety of little ways to cut back on sodium is the key. The following Take Action Today steps will help you do just that!

Take Action Today

Buy frozen or fresh vegetables instead of canned. If you do buy canned, drain the liquid off the vegetables and rinse with fresh water before cooking.

Boil water for pasta and vegetables without adding salt. Just as a watched pot never boils, adding salt doesn't make the water boil more quickly.

Always taste food before automatically salting it.

Compare the sodium level of frozen entrées and dinners. Buy those with the lowest fat and sodium levels. Combine frozen entrées with fresh fruit, breads, and milk to balance the sodium content of the whole meal.

If you use salt in cooking, try salt-free seasonings at the table.

Experiment with new and different spices. Try cinnamon on pork, fresh mint with corn, and garlic and lemon on salads.

Purchase reduced-sodium soups and tomato sauces when using them as ingredients.

Remove salt shakers from the cooking and eating areas. Replace them with salt substitutes or your own personally created spice blends.

Grandma Called It Roughage

No matter what you call it, fiber is a bigger nutrition concern than most people realize. Why? Because most people get only half the 20 to 35 grams of fiber they need each day.

Fiber has many health benefits. Because you're trying to limit your chance of getting heart disease, you need to know that eating more fiber can help lower your cholesterol levels. This is especially true of soluble fiber, found in foods such as oats, apples, carrots, and legumes. People who eat more fiber also have lower risk for certain cancers. As you cut back on fat for weight control, you may feel hungrier at times. This is because fat gives you satiety—a feeling of fullness. The great thing about fiber is that it gives you the same feeling. By eating more fiber while at the same time choosing lower-fat foods, you can prevent hunger from striking too often.

Eating more fiber is easier than you may think. The Fiber Facts chart on page 122 shows that many different foods have fiber. Using this chart as a resource, look back over your last 3 days of food records and complete the Fiber Finder below. Track the grams of fiber for each day's meals and snacks. Calculate your daily average fiber grams. Are you in the 20 to 35 gram range?

Fiber Finder

TAKE ACTION TODAY

	GRAMS OF FIBER
Day 1	
Day 2	
Day 3	
Total	
	÷ 3
Average	

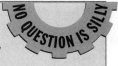

I've been trying to get more fiber by eating dried beans and peas. But I'm frustrated with how long preparing them takes—the overnight soaking and the cooking. Any suggestions on how to speed up the process?

Finding meals that are healthy and yet easy to prepare is a common frustration for today's busy families. One of the easiest ways to have dried beans and peas without all the fuss is to purchase the canned variety. Great northern, pinto, navy, and garbanzo beans are just a few that are available canned. All you have to do is open the can, drain and rinse the beans, and presto, they're ready to add to your favorite chili, pasta salad, or casserole recipe.

If your average fell below 20 grams, consider setting action steps in upcoming weeks to increase your fiber. The best sources are fruits and vegetables with edible seeds or their skins on, whole-grain breads, high-fiber cereals, and dried beans, peas, and legumes. Lettuce and popcorn, two foods thought to be high in fiber, are actually low. A few tricks for bumping up your fiber are to mix 1/4 cup of a high-fiber cereal (10 to 20 grams) with your favorite breakfast cereal, sprinkle wheat bran on the top of casseroles, or make three-bean chili instead of the version with meat. Look for food labels with "good source of fiber" listed on the front to automatically know you're getting a fiber-potent product.

Although it's tempting just to pop a pill to get the fiber you need, it's always better to get nutrients from foods. Foods that are high in fiber also have many other nutrients your body needs. For example, some fruits and vegetables contain vitamin C and beta-carotene, antioxidant vitamins that may prevent heart disease. Fiber and all these important nutrients are the added bonuses you get from eating foods.

One precaution to take when focusing on fiber is to gradually increase the number of high-fiber foods you eat. If you eat too much too soon, you'll run into trouble—abdominal cramps and constipation or diarrhea. That's enough to turn you off of fiber forever! So slowly add more fiber to your food plan and increase the amount of water you drink along with it.

As With All Things, Moderation

Have you heard of the "French Paradox?" It's the idea that drinking 1 to 2 glasses of red wine a day may lower your risk of heart disease. As a person with diabetes, you're likely to be interested when this topic comes up in

Fiber Facts

FOOD	AMOUNT	FIBER (gm)
Beans		
Baked beans, canned	1/2 cup	5-10
Black beans, cooked	1/2 cup	4
Great northern beans, cooked	1/2 cup	5
Navy Beans, cooked	1/2 cup	5
Cereals		
All-Bran	1/2 cup	10-16
Grape Nuts	1/2 cup	7
Oatmeal, cooked	1/2 cup	3
Raisin Bran	1 cup	5-7
Shredded Wheat	2 biscuits	4-5
Fruits and vegetables		
Apple, with skin	1 medium	3
Banana	1 medium	2
Grapes, red or green	1 1/2 cups	3
Orange	1 medium	3
Strawberries, fresh	1 cup	3
Raspberries, fresh	1 cup	6
Prunes, dried	3	3
Raisins	1/2 cup	3
Watermelon	2 cups	1
Potato, baked with skin	1 medium	3
Sweet potato, baked with skin	1 medium	4
Carrot, raw	1 medium	2
Brussels sprouts, cooked	1/2 cup	3
Bell pepper, raw	1/2 cup	2
Green beans, cooked	1 cup	2
Lettuce	1 cup	1
Grains		
Whole-wheat pasta, cooked	1 cup	4
Barley, cooked	1/2 cup	4
White rice, cooked	1/2 cup	<1
White bread	1 slice	<1
Whole-wheat bread	1 slice	3
Popcorn	2 cups	1

Data Source: Nutritionist IV, version 3.0, N2 Computing

conversation. You'll do anything you can to improve your health. You may also be interested in wine and other alcoholic beverages for social reasons. Many business events, family functions, holidays, and celebrations involve wine, eggnog, and other alcoholic drinks.

Just because you have diabetes doesn't mean you can't drink alcohol. If you're in good control of your diabetes, have no health problems that alcohol could make worse (high blood pressure or nephropathy), and adjust your eating habits accordingly, you can enjoy an occasional drink. But what's an occasional drink? The American Diabetes Association recommends having no more than two drinks a day. Twelve ounces of beer, four ounces of wine, or 1 1/2 ounces of hard liquor such as whiskey, gin, or vodka is considered one drink.

If you take oral medications or insulin to help regulate your glucose levels, having alcohol could send you into a low-blood sugar reaction. Under normal circumstances, when your blood glucose drops, your liver gets the signal to turn stored carbohydrate into glucose to resupply your blood. But when you drink, your liver is too busy clearing the alcohol out of your blood to make sure you have enough glucose. For this reason, having the alcohol with a meal or snack is best. So, if you're at a cocktail party or social hour, enjoy a snack with your drink. Whatever the reason you choose to drink, doing so in moderation is the healthiest choice.

If you're not really a drinker anyway, just don't feel like drinking, or are working hard to have good control of your diabetes, there are many non-alcoholic choices that are still festive. Try mineral water with a lemon or lime twist, fruit juice with carbonated water, nonalcoholic beer or wine, a "virgin" Bloody Mary, or hot cider spiced with cinnamon, cloves, and a dash of cranberry juice. Whether your drinks contain alcohol or not, always include them in your food plan and count the calories they contribute. Even though drinks are fat-free, the calories in drinks add up quickly—something to consider in your weight management plan. Alcoholic drinks don't really fit into one of the food groups, but juices used as mixers can be counted as servings from the fruit and vegetable group.

One a Day Keeps the Doctor Away?

The vitamin and mineral supplement industry has grown to be a multibillion-dollar business. But does that mean you should be popping a vitamin and mineral supplement every day? Not necessarily. If you eat a wide variety of foods, you're getting the vitamins and minerals you need for good health. Yet there are several vitamins and minerals that may interest you because of their role in diabetes, weight management, and heart disease. Here's the latest word on them.

Antioxidant vitamins. Vitamins E and C and beta-carotene are getting a lot of press these days because of their potential role in lowering the risk of heart disease. Several major research studies have found that people who take high doses of these nutrients are less likely to suffer from heart disease. Vitamin E appears to be the most beneficial. Does this mean you should take it? Not yet. No one knows if taking high doses of these vitamins may cause harm over the years. Your best strategy for now is to try to eat more foods that are packed with these vitamins. Although leafy greens do contain vitamin E, most of the food sources—nuts, seeds, vegetable oils—are also high in fat. Citrus fruits, kiwi, peppers, and broccoli are good sources of vitamin C. Beta-carotene is found in dark green and orange vegetables and fruits such as cantaloupe, sweet potatoes, and spinach.

Chromium. You may have heard that a chromium deficiency can affect your blood glucose levels. The obvious question, then, is whether a chromium supplement will give you better control of blood glucose. In reality, the majority of people with diabetes have normal chromium levels, and supplementation isn't beneficial. Anytime you're getting 1,500 calories or lower, however, you're at risk for not getting adequate amounts of all the vitamins and minerals you need for good health. Choosing foods from all the food groups will ensure that you're getting what you need. Food sources of chromium include American cheese, wheat germ, and liver.

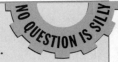

I like to eat all-natural foods. I've seen many low- and no-fat foods at the grocery store, and I'm curious if any of the fat substitutes used in these products are natural.

Actually, most of the fat substitutes used today are natural. Fat substitutes are made from protein or carbohydrate. In the protein-based fat substitutes, protein is broken down into millions of very small particles to give the slippery, creamy feel of fat in your mouth. The carbohydrate-based fat substitutes are mostly fibers that bind water to give the texture of fat. Some of the new fat substitutes are made of a non-digestible fat, giving the characteristics and taste of fat, but not the calories.

Chromium picolinate, a nutrient similar to chromium, has a variety of rumored benefits—among them improved athletic performance and weight loss. But these rumors haven't been proven true. Taking large amounts of any one mineral may, in fact, be dangerous. This habit can lead to problems with the absorption of other nutrients, and if taken in high dosages for long periods of time, some minerals can be toxic to your body. Remember, there is no magic pill for weight loss. Maintain the healthy lifestyle habits you've developed for success in weight management.

Magnesium is involved with normal glucose metabolism and heart function, and low blood levels of this mineral can increase your risk of high blood pressure or an irregular heartbeat. Good food sources of magnesium are peanut butter, tofu, shrimp, whole-grain breads, dry beans and peas, broccoli, and spinach. If your eating plan includes fewer than 1,500 calories daily, if you have a history of poor control of your diabetes, or if you're taking a diuretic on a regular basis, talk to your health care provider about the benefits of a magnesium supplement. If you have kidney disease, you shouldn't take one.

Calcium. Although there's much controversy about this theory, it's possible that persons with diabetes are at higher risk for osteoporosis (brittle bones). In general, women get osteoporosis more often than do men. When cutting back on calories to manage weight, many people choose fewer servings from the dairy group and may not get the calcium they need to prevent osteoporosis. The Recommended Dietary Allowance for calcium is 800 mg. daily, and the Daily Value on the food label recommends 1,000 mg. But other sources suggest getting even more calcium than this, up to 1,500 mg. Each day, make sure you get at least 800 mg. of calcium, and whenever possible add extra calcium-rich foods to your meal plan. The best sources of calcium are milk (1 cup = 300 mg.) and other dairy products. Look for the lowest-fat choices to get calcium with the lowest number of calories and fat grams. Although certain vegetables, such as broccoli and kale, do contain calcium, you'd need to eat up to 20 cups to get your daily requirement. If you aren't fond of milk or other dairy products, or are lactose intolerant, try taking a calcium supplement or over-the-counter antacid (most of which have calcium as their main ingredient).

It's easy to believe that any one of these supplements could be a magic bullet, the cure-all for diabetes, weight management, and heart disease. But before taking any medication—vitamin and mineral supplements included—talk to your health care provider. He or she may be able to determine if you need to take any of these nutrients, explain the side effects of the various supplements, recommend appropriate doses, and determine if the supplements interact with any medications you're currently taking.

Put One Food in Front of the Other

In this chapter you've gained a lot of knowledge about nutrition that can be useful in your personal weight and diabetes management plan. But it can seem overwhelming, too. Suddenly you're not sure if saturated fat is more important than the calorie tracking you've been doing for weight management or if you should really focus on fiber.

What you need to do is prioritize. If you have high blood pressure, spend time identifying high-sodium foods that you commonly eat and find replacements for them. But if you don't have high blood pressure, sodium may go to the bottom of your worry list. Review the topics discussed in this chapter and make a priority listing that fits your lifestyle and goals. At your next clinic visit, review this list with your health care provider. He or she knows your medical history and can help you distinguish between the issues you need to be concerned with and those you don't.

Whatever you do, don't let this new information overwhelm you and prevent you from maintaining the positive habits you've already developed. If you're counting fat grams and calories and are satisfied with your progress, continue with your current plan. You can always come back to these nutrition factors when you have questions or think it's time to tackle more issues.

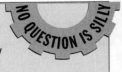

Even though this book says that margarine is better for me than butter, I've heard otherwise. I've read that margarine has trans fatty acids that turn to plastic in my arteries.

In hydrogenation, liquid oils are turned into the solid spread called margarine. During this process, the oil becomes higher in saturated fats, some of which are called trans fatty acids. It's true that trans fatty acids are more likely than liquid oils to cause buildup in your arteries, but the American Heart Association still says that saturated fat causes even more damage than trans fatty acids. You want to cut back on total fat, but when you do use fat, the best choice is a liquid oil, then margarine, and last butter.

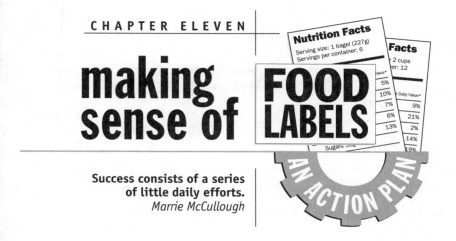

making sense of FOOD LABELS

Success consists of a series of little daily efforts.
Marrie McCullough

A great tool for anyone trying to build healthful habits is the Nutrition Facts food label. Found on virtually every food package, it's loaded with useful information to help you fine-tune your meal plan. Whether you're counting calories or fat grams, trying to get less sodium or more fiber, the information you need is all listed in plain view right on the label.

The label has been improved over the past several years, but there are still some tricks to understanding exactly which pieces of information are the best to use and what the numbers really mean. This chapter will introduce you to the food label and highlight the areas you should spend most of your time reading. So grab a label and start reading.

Label Basics

As a person with diabetes who is trying to lose weight, you may think there are just two numbers on the label that you need to know—fat and calories. There are, however, many other useful categories to consider as well.

Serving size. This is an invaluable tool in managing weight and diabetes. The nutrition information reflected on the label is per portion, and the serving size tells you how much you can eat for the fat or calorie amount listed. If the serving size listed is 1 cup but you usually eat 2 cups of the product, double the calories and fat grams to know how much you're actually getting. Serving sizes are now listed in common household measures—cups, tablespoons, or number of items (such as crackers) instead of ounces.

All brands of the same product (Peter Rabbit Canned Carrots and Bugs Bunny Canned Carrots, for example) must use the same serving size. This makes it easier for you to compare the nutritional value of different brands, without having to carry your calculator to the supermarket. Be forewarned, serving sizes on the food label may be slightly different than portions given in the Food Guide Pyramid.

Servings per container. Again, tune into this line on the label to gauge how much of the product you are actually eating. If you usually eat the whole can of soup and there are 2 servings listed on the label, be sure to adjust your calorie and fat budget accordingly.

Total calories and calories from fat. Whereas the total calories in 1 serving of a food are essential for you to know as you work on weight and diabetes management, calories-from-fat information isn't really useful. So ignore it. Now you have one less number to factor in when shopping for healthful food.

Total fat and saturated fat. To lose weight and control your risk of heart disease, these are the numbers you want to pay attention to. You're already limiting total fat as a part of your weight management plan. Compare similar products on the grocery store shelves to determine which one is lowest in fat. If you traditionally buy one brand, periodically check the total fat number on similar products. New low- and reduced-fat products are arriving in the supermarket every week. You might find one lower in fat that you like just as much as your regular brand. If you already have a handle on counting fat grams, advance your nutrition know-how by tracking saturated fat. Remember, saturated fat is the culprit in raising blood cholesterol levels, so you want to choose those products with the lowest possible number in this slot, too. No more than one-third of your total fat gram budget should come from saturated fat.

I've noticed folic acid is now on the food label of the bread I buy. Why?

If women get enough folic acid at the time of conception, they can reduce the risk of spina bifida and other neural tube defects in their unborn babies. Because half of all pregnancies are unplanned, folic acid is required to be added (as of Jan. 1, 1998) to all enriched products such as bread, cornmeal, and pasta to make sure women are getting enough.

Cholesterol. This number tells you the amount of cholesterol in one serving. But don't be fooled. Just because you find a zero in the cholesterol category doesn't mean the food is fat free, too. Cholesterol is found only in animal products, so foods such as vegetable oils, snack foods, and convenience products can be cholesterol free and still high in fat.

Sodium. Depending on the nutrition priorities you have set for your weight and diabetes management, and whether or not you have high blood pressure, you may need to watch this number. In general, convenience products (frozen dinners, boxed mixes, snack foods, etc.) modified to be lower in fat tend to be high in sodium. The food manufacturers have taken out the fat but put salt in for flavor. Other high-sodium foods include canned products such as soups and vegetables, luncheon meats, and certain snack foods, such as chips and nuts. The food label suggests 2,400 milligrams as a daily upper limit for sodium.

Total carbohydrate, dietary fiber, and sugars. For the first time ever, the carbohydrates in a food product have been broken down by type on the label. There are separate categories for total carbohydrate, fiber, and sugar, so that you know what type of carbohydrate you're getting. By using this information, you can more effectively balance your carbohydrates throughout the day. Try to purchase foods that are higher in fiber and total carbohydrates and lower in sugars. Although persons with diabetes can eat sugar, you still want to limit foods with lots of sugar and not much else—so-called empty-calorie foods.

Protein. Because most people get more protein than they need, this is another number you can ignore. Without even having to think about it, you're most likely getting plenty of protein. If you have renal failure as a complication of diabetes, however, you'll want to pay closer attention to the protein content of foods. Discuss an appropriate level of protein with your health care provider and dietitian.

Daily Value. The Food and Drug Administration (FDA), which is responsible for the format of the food label, concluded that the average person eats about 2,000 calories a day. Based on this calorie level, the FDA considered current healthy eating recommendations and came up with amounts of fat, saturated fat, sodium, cholesterol, total carbohydrate, and fiber that the average person would need each day. These numbers, then, make up the Daily Value and are listed in the footnote of most food labels.

The Daily Value for fat is 65 grams, for carbohydrate 300 grams, and for fiber 25 grams.

Percent Daily Value. The percent Daily Value looks at how 1 serving of a food fits into the daily allowances of the average person who eats 2,000 calories a day. For example, if a cereal has 3 fat grams in 1 cup, then 1 serving has 5 percent of the Daily Value ($3 \div 65 \times 100 = 5$ percent). One serving provides 5 percent of the fat recommended for this person on a given day. If you wanted to, you could eat 20 servings of this cereal and have reached your fat limit for the day. Because your calorie level and fat budget may vary from the assumed averages on the food label, Daily Value and percent Daily Value aren't very useful pieces of information. The absolute numbers—grams of fat and total calories per serving—are much more important to your specific eating plan.

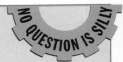

On the label for my favorite cereal, sugar isn't listed as an ingredient, but the Nutrition Facts says there are 4 grams of sugar per serving. Which is correct?

Most likely, they're both correct. Although table sugar isn't listed as an ingredient, it might be coming from a different source in the food. Raisins and other dried fruits would contribute some sugar. Honey, corn syrup, or dextrose are other names for sugar that you might notice in the ingredient declaration. The sugar number given in the Nutrition Facts panel takes into account all these various forms.

Facts at a Glance

Today's labeling regulations make it possible, at a glance, to see that certain products are healthier choices—without having to read the entire Nutrition Facts food label. Nutrient content claims and health claims are ways for food manufacturers to highlight this information for you on the front of the label so that you can make healthier choices with a quick glance at the grocery store shelf.

There are three kinds of nutrient content claims: absolute, relative (or comparative), and implied. Low fat is an example of an absolute claim because it tells you exactly how much of a nutrient is in one serving of the food. A low-fat product can have no more than 3 fat grams per serving. Other examples of absolute claims are:

fat free less than 0.5 grams per serving

low cholesterol less than 20 milligrams per serving

low sodium less than 140 milligrams per serving

low calorie less than 40 calories per serving

lean less than 10 grams fat, 4 grams saturated fat, and 95 milligrams cholesterol per serving

extra lean less than 5 grams fat, 2 grams saturated fat, and 95 milligrams cholesterol per serving

good source contains 10 to 19 percent of the Daily Value for a nutrient (such as fiber or vitamin C)

Relative, or comparative, claims compare the amount of a nutrient in a food with the amount of the same nutrient in another food. For example, a reduced-fat blueberry muffin would have 25 percent less fat than a regular blueberry muffin. Other comparative claims are:

light or lite contains one-third fewer calories or one-half the fat

more or added contains at least 10 percent more of the Daily Value of a nutrient (such as calcium or fiber)

The third type of nutrient content claim, an implied claim, is more subjective. Because you would expect a product whose package says "high in oat bran" to have a lot of fiber, the food must meet the definition of a "good source" of fiber.

Health claims are different than nutrient claims because health claims talk about the relationship between a nutrient and a specific disease. Not getting enough calcium can lead to osteoporosis (brittle bones), so foods that are a good source of calcium can claim that their product may help reduce the risk of this disease. Other health claims you may see on a food label relate low-fat foods and fruits and vegetables to a reduced risk of cancer, low-sodium foods to a lowered risk of high blood pressure, or folic acid to reducing a woman's risk of having a child with a brain or spinal-cord defect.

Although nutrient content and health claims provide valuable information to consumers, you should realize that just because a product doesn't list a claim doesn't mean it isn't good for you. There are many products that meet the definition of "low fat" but just don't make this claim on the front of the label. Salsas are a good example. Because they're all fat free, you'll rarely see this highlighted on the label. Fat-free salsa isn't new or different, so food manufacturers choose not to waste the space for this message on the label. So even though claims make your job of hunting for healthful foods easier, you'll still need to turn the package around and read the Nutrition Facts food label.

How Do You Label an Orange?

It doesn't come in a package, it's relatively small in size, and no two are quite the same, so how do you label an orange? Or, for that matter, how do you label any fruit or vegetable in the produce section? What about fresh seafood in the refrigerated case?

Because it isn't practical to label them directly, you won't find the Nutrition Facts on fresh fruits and vegetables. Supermarkets are required, however, to provide shoppers with nutrition information on the 20 most popular fruits and vegetables. Look for signs in the produce section that tell you the nutritional value of the fruit or vegetable, or find this information in brochures or on the package itself if this is practical (with pre-cut lettuce salads, for example). The same rule applies to the top 20 fresh fish and seafoods.

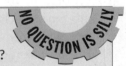

The right-hand column on a food label says it has 20 percent fat. With 13 fat grams and 300 calories, I calculate 39 percent fat. Am I figuring something wrong?

No, you're not. The number on the label just means something different than you think it means. The right-hand column of numbers is the % Daily Value. These percentages tell you how 1 serving of this food fits into a 2,000-calorie eating plan, which the label assumes is the right amount for the average person. This person would be allowed 65 fat grams per day. Thirteen divided by 65 gives you 20 percent of the Daily Value for fat. On the other hand, you're calculating the percent of calories from fat in 1 serving of this food, which is 39 percent. A much easier way for you to use food labels is to remember your personal daily fat gram budget and determine how each food fits into it.

You Won't Find a Label Here

Although the vast majority of foods will carry the Nutrition Facts food label, there are certain products that you won't be able to find a label on anywhere. These include

foods that have no nutritional value such as spices, coffee, and tea

foods made in the deli or bakery of a grocery store

foods in very small packages, such as those sold in vending machines

restaurant foods

foods produced by small companies

medical foods

The category that deserves further explanation is restaurant foods. Because the average person spends half of his or her food dollars eating out, taking out, or driving through, it would be beneficial to have nutrition information available for restaurant foods. But you can imagine how difficult this would be for restaurants. To satisfy their customers, restaurants change their menus frequently and offer various specials. Many restaurants take special orders and requests. Suppliers of restaurant ingredients change frequently. All these factors make labeling these foods very difficult.

So restaurants, hospital cafeterias, cafeterias in worksites, and similar operations are not required to give the nutrition information on their menu items. This all changes, however, if they make a claim (call their veggie burger "low fat," for example). If they choose to say their food item has a special nutrition quality, then they have to provide nutrition information to the customer. This doesn't mean you'll find it all spelled out on the menu, but the information must be kept in the establishment so that it can at least be verbally passed on to you.

Although restaurants are not required to provide nutrition information, you'll find that eating out has gotten easier for the health-conscious diner. Many restaurants, especially fast-food places and national chains, do have nutrition information available in a brochure. Even mom-and-pop shops are clueing in to the nutrition trend by either highlighting the healthier options on their menu (with an apple or a heart, for example) or listing the pertinent nutrition facts along with the menu description.

The True Test: Are You Label Able?

Use the label below to test your knowledge of what is and isn't important on the food label for weight and diabetes management. On the sample shown, circle the three most important numbers for you to check when you're grocery shopping and cross out three numbers that you can ignore on the label.

Nutrition Facts

Serving size: 1 slice (227g)
Servings per container: 1

Amount per serving

Calories 220 **Calories from Fat** 30

% Daily Value*

Total Fat 3g	**5%**
Saturated Fat 2g	**10%**
Cholesterol 20mg	**7%**
Sodium 135mg	**6%**
Total Carbohydrate 38g	**13%**
Dietary Fiber 0g	**0%**
Sugars 38g	
Protein 10g	

Vitamin A 2%	•	Vitamin C 0%
Calcium 35%	•	Iron 0%

* Percent Daily Values are based on a 2,000 calorie diet. Your daily values may be higher or lower depending on your calorie needs.

If you circled serving size, calories, carbohydrate, fat grams, or saturated fat as crucial pieces of information, you're correct. If you crossed out % Daily Value, calories from fat, cholesterol, or protein (unless you have kidney disease), you're a labeling genius.

As you can tell, a lot of information is packed into the Nutrition Facts food label. Although each part of the food label is important, you personally don't need to check every line to be successful in weight and diabetes management. Reality is, you probably don't have the time to scrutinize every aspect of the label on your weekly shopping trips. Once you've identified some products you like, you can check less frequently, and then only for new products.

special occasions made easy

If there's a way to do it better...find it.
Thomas A. Edison

AN ACTION PLAN

Up to this point, you may have limited yourself from eating out or attending social gatherings. You might be saying to yourself, "I can't eat out, everything's too high in fat." While it's true that special occasions often revolve around food, at least most are predictable. You enjoy the same goodies during the winter holiday season, for example, or salads on the Fourth of July. The key is planning ahead, learning how to make wise food choices, and sticking with your exercise routine.

In this chapter, you'll take a look at your current social eating habits, master the art of maintaining good blood glucose control when eating away from home, develop skills necessary for interpreting the menu maze, and create specific, realistic action plans designed to help you continue to achieve your health goals every day—special occasion or not.

Restaurant Eating, Made to Order

Before you can make changes, you must first evaluate your current social eating patterns. If you're like most people, eating out is a normal part of day-to-day living—it's not just for special occasions such as birthdays or anniversaries anymore. In fact, you may eat as many as one of every three meals away from home. You might be thinking, "I don't eat out that much." It all depends on how you define eating out. Think about it. If you were to grab a muffin with that mug of coffee at the coffee shop, eat a sandwich from the cafeteria at work, and pick up a pizza on the way home from work, that would be three meals eaten out. Amazing, isn't it? In today's fast-paced world, it's easy to do without ever really thinking about it.

So take a minute now to analyze your dining habits. Complete the Eating Away From Home Work Sheet below. If you're still keeping track of what you eat using the Fat and Calorie Control Work Sheet from chapter 3, you have what you need for this exercise. If not, take time now to start recording what you eat again. This will help you gain a better understanding of what choices you make, how often you eat out, and where you eat your meals.

Eating Away From Home Work Sheet

Answer the following questions using your food records. Once you've completed the work sheet, read on to see how making a few changes in your habits can add up to a big difference in your diabetes and weight management plan.

1. I typically eat meals out or away from home at

breakfast	times per week
lunch	times per week
dinner	times per week

2. The places I generally eat include

❏ coffee shops   ❏ delicatessens   ❏ work cafeterias
❏ family-style restaurants   ❏ vending machines   ❏ fine dining
❏ takeout (Chinese, pizza)

3. I order or select the following foods:

_____

_____

4. I choose the following beverages:

_____

_____

5. My meal times   ❏ vary   ❏ stay about the same

6. I eat until   ❏ slightly hungry   ❏ satisfied   ❏ stuffed

Dining Out Without Doing Your Diabetes In

Your main goal when eating away from home is to maintain the habits you've built to manage your weight and diabetes. It's easy to let new lifestyle habits get tossed aside when celebrating special occasions such as birthdays or anniversaries. But with a little planning, you can still dine out and maintain your food plan for diabetes management. Here are a few strategies to help you maintain control whether you're eating at a restaurant, work party, or family gathering.

Plan ahead. Think about the number of days you indicated you eat out on the previous work sheet. Did you note how many calories and fat grams you had left for the day so that you could eat accordingly? Because it's extremely easy to eat higher-fat foods when dining out, plan to eat low-fat or fat-free foods before and after your restaurant meal so that you can stay within your fat gram budget. On weeks when dining out is more frequent than usual, reduce your fat grams by 5 to 10 a day whenever possible.

Adjust mealtimes to maintain consistent eating patterns. When you eat out, do your mealtimes vary or stay about the same? For best blood glucose control, eat at your regularly scheduled mealtime—especially if you take any type of medication for your diabetes. If you're eating about 1 hour later than usual, have a snack (such as fruit or crackers) at your normal eating time and then follow with your meal. If you expect your mealtime to be delayed for more than an hour, swap meal and snack times. For example, if you typically eat a bedtime snack, eat your snack at your regularly scheduled mealtime and your meal later. Maintaining your routine helps to regulate blood glucose levels.

Practice portion control. It's easy to get distracted when socializing with others and unconsciously snack on the bread basket or salad bar before the meal and still eat all of your entrée. Make a special effort to track how much you're eating. If you're starting to feel full, ask for food to be packaged to bring home or have your plate removed from the table.

Balance your food choices. As you know, monitoring the number of carbohydrate choices you eat at each meal is essential for maintaining blood glucose levels. Look back to your answers on the Eating Away From Home Work Sheet. What types of food and beverage choices do you typically make at restaurants? Foods such as milk, fruits, and breads have the greatest effect on blood glucose. That's why it's important to continue eating the same number of servings from these groups at meals—even those eaten away from home. If there isn't much fruit on the menu, or you didn't have milk, feel free to eat another bread serving or a larger portion of pasta or rice. Consistency is the key no matter where you're eating.

Restaurant Eating the Low-Fat Way

Now that you know the basics of controlling your diabetes when eating away from home, it's time to learn the ins and outs of low-fat eating in these same situations. Staying on track with your meal plan can be challenging at restaurants, but with some strategies and a positive "I can do it" attitude, maintaining healthful habits is manageable.

Consider the following Take Action Today strategies to help you stay within your fat gram budget and find the best picks on any restaurant menu. Use these as action steps in the upcoming weeks when you know you'll be eating out.

Take Action Today Tips

Call ahead. Sticking to your health goals begins even before you arrive at the restaurant. If you call ahead, you'll know what menu choices are available and can decide what you'll eat before you leave home. That way you won't be tempted by high-calorie, high-fat menu options or by what other people are ordering.

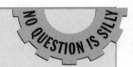

When I go out to eat, I generally choose some type of salad and have one or two alcoholic drinks. Do the drinks negate my healthy salad choice?

It's true that salad greens are low in calories; however, cheese, croutons, nuts and seeds, and regular salad dressings make many salads high in fat and calories. Opt for salads packed with vegetables and topped with low-fat or fat-free dressings.

As for the alcohol, it doesn't negate healthful food choices, but it doesn't add any nutritional value to your meal either. Occasionally having alcohol is fine, but keep in mind that it will impact your blood glucose levels (refer to discussion on alcohol in chapter 10). Avoid drinks such as liqueurs and cordials that are high calorie due to their sugar content.

Inspect the menu. Although you may feel embarrassed or nervous about asking lots of questions, you shouldn't. Your health is important. So know exactly what you're getting. Ask for a clear explanation of ingredients and preparation methods.

Recognize fat-laden foods. To combat fat, skip fried and sautéed foods and any menu items prepared breaded, batter dipped, creamed, or au gratin. Stay clear of Alfredo, béarnaise, and hollandaise sauces, too.

Know low-fat terms. Savor the flavor of menu items prepared baked, broiled, poached, steamed, roasted, or grilled. Enjoy lean red meats, skinless poultry, seafood, pasta with red sauces, and vegetable salads with vinaigrette or low-fat salad dressings.

Understand menu lingo. Think twice about choices like "diet plates" that consist of a beef patty and cottage cheese or vegetarian dishes loaded with nuts and cheese. They aren't always the most nutritious choices and can be high in fat.

You should also know that restaurants need to follow the same guidelines as food companies when they use terms such as "low fat" or "reduced calorie." When you see these terms, the restaurant must provide the nutrition information for the item you're ordering.

Make special requests. Check to see if certain items can be served in a healthier manner. Does the vegetable of the day already have butter on it, or could it be served plain? Is skim or low-fat milk available? Can the bread basket be brought with the meal? If this will keep you from eating too much before your entrée arrives, ask!

Eat slowly. Experience the taste and texture of the food, the atmosphere, and the conversation and appreciate the luxury of dining out.

Tune in to body signals. Are you still physically hungry? Or are you eating without paying attention to how you feel? The goal is to stop eating when you're still comfortable, not when you're stuffed. Once you've eaten until satisfied, request that your food be packaged to take home so that you don't keep nibbling.

Understand your ethnic foods. Most ethnic restaurants offer a wide variety of menu options. Enjoy stir-fried foods without breading or deep-fried meats. Ask that Mexican foods be served without all the cheese, sour cream, and guacamole. Choose pastas with vegetable-based sauces and

A Banquet of Many Nations

GRAINS

Enjoy 6–11 servings daily—Chinese: cellophane noodles, rice, rice congee (rice soup), rice sticks (rice flour noodles), rice vermicelli (thin rice pasta); **Italian:** bread sticks, gnocchi (dumpling), Italian bread, linguine, polenta (cornmeal mush), risotto, spaghetti; **Mexican:** cooked rice, corn tortilla (soft), crackers, flour tortilla (soft), posole (soup made with corn kernels), sopa (thick rice soup), taco shell; **Vegetarian:** bulgur, couscous, rice, wheat berries, wheat germ

FRUITS

Enjoy 2–4 servings daily—Chinese: apple, guava, kumquat, lychee nuts, oranges, persimmon, star fruit; **Italian:** blueberries, dried figs, grapefruit, pomegranate, raspberries; **Mexican:** apple, avocado, mango, papaya, plantano (cooking banana), zapote (sweet yellowish fruit); **Vegetarian:** fresh fruit, fruit juices

VEGETABLES

Enjoy 3–5 servings daily—Chinese: baby corn, bamboo shoots, broccoli, pea pods, straw mushrooms, yard long beans; **Italian:** artichoke, eggplant, green or red pepper, marinara sauce, mushrooms, spinach; **Mexican:** chayote (Mexican squash), corn, jicama (root vegetable), tomato, nopales (cactus leaves); **Vegetarian:** bamboo shoots, bean sprouts, raw vegetables, vegetable juices

MEAT, POULTRY, FISH, AND DRY BEANS

Enjoy 2–3 servings daily—Chinese: steamed chicken, fish, lobster, pork, scallops, shrimp, or tofu; **Italian:** beans, beef, chicken, fish, lentils, steamed clams or mussels, squid, veal; **Mexican:** beans, beef, chicken; **Vegetarian:** beans, falafel, humus, tempeh, tofu, vegetarian burgers

DAIRY PRODUCTS

Enjoy 2–3 servings daily—Chinese: fortified soy cheese, fortified soy milk, milk; **Italian:** gelato, milk, mozzarella cheese, ricotta cheese, yogurt; **Mexican:** custard, leche (milk); **Vegetarian:** fortified soy cheese, fortified soy milk, goat milk, yogurt

FATS, OILS, AND SWEETS

Use sparingly—Chinese: hoisin sauce, oyster sauce, soy sauce; **Italian:** butter, chocolate, heavy whipping cream, Italian ice, olive oil, olives, pine nuts; **Mexican:** butter, candy, fried pork rinds, guacamole, sour cream; **Vegetarian:** avocados, nuts, olives, seeds, tahini

A Banquet of Many Nations (continued)

BEST PICKS: COMBINATION FOODS

Chinese: mu shu vegetables, steamed dumplings or dim sum with chicken, stir-fried chicken or beef with vegetables, vegetable or chicken lo mein; **Italian:** chicken cacciatore, cioppino, chicken marsala (no skin), minestrone soup, pasta e faioli, pasta with marinara sauce (no meat), pasta primavera, linguini with red clam sauce; **Mexican:** arroz con pollo (chicken with rice, no skin), fajitas, soft chicken taco with lettuce and tomato, soft bean, vegetable, or fish burrito (no refried beans or cheese), chicken, seafood, or bean enchiladas with green sauce or hot sauce (no cheese, sour cream, or guacamole); **Vegetarian:** bean or lentil soups, vegetables curries, basmati rice with vegetables or saffron, bean burritos (no cheese or sour cream)

grilled meats—no sausage. Select vegetarian meals packed with steamed or grilled vegetables prepared without cheese or nuts. Refer to A Banquet of Many Nations for more ideas on healthful choices at common ethnic restaurants.

Enjoy all foods in moderation. If you really love chocolate-turtle cheesecake, ask someone to share a piece with you. Splurging once in a while on a higher-fat item is not a problem for most people.

Eating out is a great way to enjoy dishes you wouldn't generally prepare at home, a means of relaxation or entertainment, a chance to experience the foods and flavors of different cultures, an opportunity to get a break from the kids, the dirty dishes, or the office. Most important, it's a wonderful way to mix the joy of eating with the company of family and friends. So enjoy the company, the atmosphere, and healthful, flavorful food. Making smart food choices no matter where you are is an important step toward improving your health.

Eat Fast, Not Fat

It's the grab 'n' go generation, with one-fourth of most meals eaten away from home at fast-food restaurants. Not surprising. Fast-food chains are everywhere—shopping malls, hospitals, high school cafeterias, and street corners. People head for these quick and convenient restaurants to save time. But how do fast foods fit into your health plan? It's no secret that most are high in calories and laden with fat and sodium. If you're not careful, the convenience of quick dining may eat up your fat gram budget for the day and throw off your blood glucose levels.

If I choose lower-fat menu options, can I eat as much as I want?

NO QUESTION IS SILLY

As you know, eating low fat is an integral part of your weight management plan. However, keep in mind that when you eat out, you usually receive generous portions of foods. If you eat large quantities of low-fat foods, you can still get too many calories. Eating larger portions at any one meal can also throw off your blood glucose control. So in addition to choosing low-fat foods, be consistent with portions and try to listen to your body's internal cues—the ones that tell you when you're satisfied (full), but not stuffed.

So what's a realistic fast-food meal? How many fat grams can you eat at any one meal? Can you keep blood glucose levels in control? To maintain your diabetes management and weight, let the food pyramid help you. Eat a consistent number of servings from the fruit, milk, and bread groups. Refer back to the Fat and Calorie Control Work Sheets you've been using to see how many servings you typically eat from each group. Then refer to The Fast and Healthy Food Pyramid (page 143) to make your fast-food choices—trying to maintain your typical pattern of eating. Because fruit and vegetable choices are often limited, bring fresh fruit or vegetable sticks from home to round out your meal.

Making choices from The Fast and Healthy Food Pyramid will also keep you on track with your fat gram budget. It's designed to help you single out the lower-fat choices. The goal is to use no more than one-third to one-half of your fat budget for the day when eating at a fast-food restaurant. To do this, your choices should be heavier toward the bottom of the pyramid and leaner at the top. When you make choices from the bottom, remember to make these low-fat as well. For example, choose soft-shell instead of hard-shell tacos or a hamburger bun instead of a croissant or biscuit sandwich. Limit items from the top of the pyramid, such as deep-fried or breaded items, bacon, regular salad dressings, special sauces, and mayonnaise. Share cookies or an apple turnover with a friend occasionally.

For specific fat gram information on a variety of fast-food choices, refer to appendix A. You should note that this table isn't all-inclusive. Items at fast-food restaurants change quickly. To get an updated listing, ask the restaurant at your next visit. Most have nutrition information readily available.

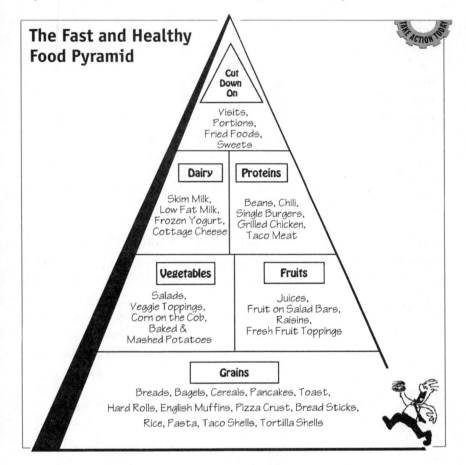

The Fast and Healthy Food Pyramid

Cut Down On
Visits, Portions, Fried Foods, Sweets

Dairy
Skim Milk, Low Fat Milk, Frozen Yogurt, Cottage Cheese

Proteins
Beans, Chili, Single Burgers, Grilled Chicken, Taco Meat

Vegetables
Salads, Veggie Toppings, Corn on the Cob, Baked & Mashed Potatoes

Fruits
Juices, Fruit on Salad Bars, Raisins, Fresh Fruit Toppings

Grains
Breads, Bagels, Cereals, Pancakes, Toast, Hard Rolls, English Muffins, Pizza Crust, Bread Sticks, Rice, Pasta, Taco Shells, Tortilla Shells

TAKE ACTION TODAY

Surviving Social Gatherings and Holidays

Although you might find managing your blood glucose levels and making low-fat food choices is getting easier when you dine out, it's those once-a-year holidays and special occasions that frequently detour your new health habits. It can be hard to maintain a positive attitude and manage stress during busy holidays—let alone stick with your new food and activity habits.

Undeniably, holidays and special occasions such as weddings are fun and important occasions. They're times when friends and family members get together to renew old ties and make new ones. But they can also present a challenge. Too many high-fat, high-calorie treats, along with decreased physical activity, can lead to weight gain. They can also present a challenge for diabetes control. No matter what the occasion, you need to continue to practice the strategies discussed earlier in the chapter for improved blood glucose management.

So how can you enjoy each event and continue to maintain health habits? The key is to determine your strategy early and write an action plan for success. Health doesn't just happen. You need to plan action steps consistent with your diabetes and weight management goals. In the next section, you'll walk through the steps and learn how to complete the Surviving Special Occasions Work Sheet. Use this form for each individual special event that comes up throughout the year. As you review the following steps, record your answers under the corresponding question on the work sheet (page 147).

Step 1: Assess Potential Detours in Maintaining Health Habits

When you know a special occasion is coming up, take time to define how the special occasion makes it difficult for you to stick with your health goals. It could be that no low-fat options are available or that it's hard to be active when you're away from home. Record your answers under the first question on the work sheet. If the special occasion triggers overeating, refer back to chapter 7 and use the Break the Chain Activity work sheet.

Step 2: List Potential Strategies to Overcome Barriers

Depending on where your difficulties lie, you may have strategies on how to stick with your food plan, increase your activity level, or reduce the stress that is sometimes associated with special occasions. You may want to refer back to the many Take Action Today tips from other chapters for additional ideas.

One example of a strategy to stick with your food plan could be calling the host of a holiday party to ask what is being served, offer to bring a side dish, or ask questions. Although at first calling may feel uncomfortable, keep in mind that if you were allergic to peanuts and had severe reactions from eating them, you wouldn't hesitate to ask questions, would you? It may be true that sticking to your fat and calorie budget is not as drastic as an allergic reaction, but if it's important to you, don't underestimate it. By taking action steps to preplan, assert yourself, and listen to your internal signals of hunger and fullness, you'll be one step closer to your weight and diabetes management goals.

If maintaining your activity or exercise routine is an issue, sneak in some extra activity by playing more with children or treating the dog to an extra walk. Better yet, start a new family tradition that gets everyone moving. Plan a cross-country skiing outing, a volleyball game, or a family walk. A break from sitting and eating not only burns additional calories but renews lost energy after a big meal.

If certain special occasions really stress you out, your strategies should help you cope more effectively. Remember to take a time-out to relax in a hot bath, get in a nap, or read a book. The key is planning your strategies in advance and getting them down on paper. Once you've brainstormed some ideas, you can move to the next step.

Will my family be upset if I make a "healthy" holiday meal this year?

NO QUESTION IS SILLY

Your family will definitely not hate you, but they may resist if you suggest changing old holiday favorites. Ask them to support you in your health goals and tell them the food will still taste great—it will just be different. In fact, depending on what you traditionally prepare—you could make a few recipe modifications, such as using lower-fat cheese or less fat in recipes—they may not even notice the taste difference or that you've made the item healthier.

Step 3: Decide What Action Steps You Can Realistically Take

Look over your potential strategies again and choose one or two you can achieve. Your action steps for the day of the special occasion might be to bring a low-fat dish to the party or go for a 30-minute walk before breakfast. The actions need to be reasonable, reflecting areas of weight and diabetes management that you've already been working on. Whatever you decide, write out your plan on the work sheet or use the pages provided in chapter 6 for recording action steps. Writing your action down improves your chances of actually doing it.

Step 4: Ask for Support From Others

As you learned in chapter 8, people can sabotage or enhance your health habits. Although you may be focused on losing weight and managing your diabetes—whether it's a special occasion or not—others might be focused on past traditions. When you arrive at the summer picnic, aunt Cassie might hand you a slice of your favorite dessert, saying, "I made it for you." Or if you're trying to maintain your exercise routine, your family might tell you, "It's a holiday, you can skip exercise for a day." What can you do? Be assertive. Tell your aunt, "I appreciate your efforts to make my favorite dessert, but I'm working hard to maintain my weight and manage my diabetes. Thanks for understanding when I decline." As for the exercise, say, "I feel better about myself when I stick with my exercise routine. I know you'll understand if I need to get away from the festivities for a while to be active."

Step 5: Reward Yourself

It's important to give yourself a boost when you stick with your action plan. Reward yourself with things that reinforce behavior change such as a massage or a new CD. Avoid rewards that involve food.

Practice, Practice, Practice

No matter what the occasion, you can make choices that continuously improve your health. To adapt the skills you've learned in this chapter, review them regularly as reminders, track your fat and calorie intake using the Fat and Calorie Control Work Sheets from chapter 3 to assess how you're doing, and complete the Surviving Special Occasions Work Sheet whenever you plan to attend a family gathering, party, or those once-a-year festivities. With strategies in hand, you're destined for success.

Surviving Special Occasions Work Sheet

TAKE ACTION TODAY

Upcoming Special Occasion _____

1. This special occasion makes it difficult for me to stick with my weight and diabetes goals because

_____

_____

_____

2. Several strategies I could use to stick with my health goals are

_____

_____

_____

_____

3. My specific action steps (food, activity, and self-care) for this occasion are to

_____

_____

_____

_____

4. One way my family, friends, or coworkers can support me during this event is by

_____

_____

_____

_____

5. My reward for achieving my action steps is

_____

_____

How can I manage my time and reduce stress with so many commitments during the November-to-January holiday season?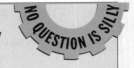

You can start by planning ahead. During the holiday season, for example, you can record every office party, church gathering, school concert, or family get-together on your calendar so that you can visualize the number of social events you could attend. Once you have them all down, prioritize them with the rest of the family to determine if there are some less important ones you could miss.

Although limiting commitments is the first place to start, next you need to review tasks to be done. You could mail close friends and relatives cards at various times during the year (instead of the holidays) and order gifts from catalogs throughout the year to avoid the holiday mall rush. Delegate tasks as well. You can ask others to buy some gifts for you, help wrap presents, or share responsibilities when preparing the big holiday meals.

CHAPTER THIRTEEN

lapse
does not equal
relapse

AN ACTION PLAN

**Our greatest glory is not in never falling,
but in rising every time we fall.**
Confucius

In chapter 7, you explored the stages of change and discovered where you are in this cycle. One additional step could be added to this cycle of change—lapse and relapse. If you've previously lost weight and then gained it all back, you've experienced lapses and relapse. Likewise if you've quit smoking and later started again. Or gotten out of credit card debt and then charged up a storm. Or even started several projects around the house and never finished them.

By following this book's action plan, you've likely gained strides toward your long-term health goal. Nothing can stop you now; you're motivated and energized about your current success. But the preceding examples— losing weight then gaining it back or smoking again—are a good reality check. Although it might not be evident right now, lapses and relapse are normal. They'll occur at some point in this journey you've embarked on. But don't get discouraged; by understanding lapses and relapse ahead of time, you'll be prepared to deal with them when they do occur and can stay in control of your new healthier habits. The goal of this chapter is to help you gain skill in preventing lapses from turning into a relapse.

Lapse Versus Relapse

To stay on track with your weight and diabetes management plan, it's essential to understand the difference between a lapse and a relapse. The simplest definition of a lapse is a slip or mistake. Consider a professional ice-skater who loses her concentration during competition and falls after a triple axle. She may have fallen, but she still has the ability to skate. She simply made a mistake. That's what makes a lapse different from a relapse—corrective action can still be taken. Complete control hasn't been lost.

In the areas of weight and diabetes management there are many examples of lapse: eating a large popcorn with butter at the movies, going several days without monitoring blood glucose levels, missing aerobics class all week, or gaining 2 pounds back.

How you respond to situations such as these determines whether they will stop at just a lapse or become a full-fledged relapse. A string of lapses together makes a relapse. When the new habits you've developed backslide into the old habits, you're experiencing relapse. Examples of when you've lost control in weight and diabetes management might include a returning to your previous weight or no longer monitoring your blood glucose levels.

What Leads to Lapses and Relapses

Although there may not seem to be a clear-cut line between lapse and relapse, various factors predict the likelihood of lapses becoming relapse. These factors are your emotional state, motivation level, coping skills, and physiological factors such as cravings, support, and social factors. As you read the following explanations, consider your personality and lifestyle to determine which factors have already or could potentially affect your success at long-term diabetes and weight management.

Your emotions. Although lapses are typically associated with situational factors such as overeating at parties or with certain people, relapses are related to emotional factors. Negative emotions such as anxiety, frustration, and depression can contribute to relapse. Stress is a major predictor, and some studies show that almost half of all relapses occur during stressful times.

Your motivation. When you've just learned that you have a chronic disease such as diabetes, your motivation is high. You're geared up to exercise, eat right, and make other changes necessary to improve your health and quality of life. This burst of enthusiasm is normal. The trick is maintaining it. Success with your long-term health goals can vary depending on whether motivation comes from external or internal sources. External sources, such as pressure from your doctor, family, or friends, won't get you through in the long run. The motivation needs to come from inside you.

Your coping skills. There are two parts to coping with lapse to prevent relapse—believing you are capable of responding to lapses and having skills readily accessible to prevent them. Creative visualization and self-talk are two coping skills you'll learn more about in chapter 14. Thinking about how you might prevent a relapse before you find yourself in the middle of one is useful. Considering how you've overcome other stressful, trying situations can also help you identify coping skills to maintain your new, healthier habits.

Your genes. More and more evidence suggests that genetics play a role in obesity. One theory—called the set-point theory—says your body will always try to revert to a heavier weight at which it was comfortable. Another idea about the role of genetics says you have a certain number of fat cells that you can't ever lower. Either way, there is definitely a component of weight that is truly beyond your control. Awareness of the idea that genetics may be an obstacle can help stop you from reverting to old habits once you've lost weight.

Support. You know by now that weight management isn't just a food issue. There are many components of this complicated disorder called being overweight. Just as these various factors can contribute to weight gain, they can contribute to weight loss. Support is a perfect example. Up to half of all relapses can be associated with conflicts with a spouse, child, parent, friend, coworker, or significant other. By the same token, strong interpersonal relationships and a solid support system can ensure success at weight and diabetes management.

I've had major swings in my weight over the past 10 years. Why should I even bother to lose weight?

NO QUESTION IS SILLY

Your frustration with weight loss is understandable, but this time it can be different. If you really focus on dealing with the minor slipups before they overwhelm you, and realize that this is a lifelong process, you can find true success in managing weight. The best reason you have now to manage your weight is the improvement you'll see in your diabetes. Living with a chronic disease is never easy, but knowing that you can control it and prevent or delay long-term complications through a healthy lifestyle can make the day-to-day reality of the disease easier.

Social factors. Whereas smokers are told to avoid cigarettes completely after kicking the habit, and recovering alcoholics never to drink another drop of alcohol, people who have weight issues can't totally avoid food. You need to eat to survive. But what you can do is limit your exposure to social situations or people that may send you from lapse into relapse. In chapter 7, you discovered the cues that trigger your overeating (people, emotions, activity, special event, sensory). Review your cues and consider minimizing those events or situations that may turn your lapse into a relapse.

It's probably obvious to you by now that each of these factors has both a positive and a negative side. They can be used either way to affect your goals. Look back and highlight the factors that are most likely to affect you personally. Consider how you can use them positively to control lapses and continue on your path of weight and diabetes management.

Developing Your Personal Prevention Plan

Weight control and diabetes management are similar in many ways to the children's game Chutes and Ladders. You take several strong steps forward, hit a chute (or a lapse), and slide back a few steps. You regain your position, move ahead, and again slide a few steps in reverse. Although you periodically experience setbacks along the way, your overall direction is forward. This is how you win the game. Controlling the lapses is what prevents a complete backslide to your original starting point.

While this sounds simple enough, the trick is to have a well thought out game plan. You need established methods of dealing with lapses before they happen. Using the five steps detailed here, prepare yourself for dealing with the slipups that are bound to occur.

Accept that you won't be perfect during your weight management journey. One day you'll eat more calories than planned or skip exercising because you just don't feel like doing it. Acknowledging up front that times like this will occur puts you in control of these situations and alters how you react when a lapse does occur. You'll view it as what it is—a lapse.

Take a time-out. When you're experiencing a lapse, try to remove yourself physically or mentally from the situation or temptation to a place where you can think rationally and objectively about the lapse. If you get anxious or frustrated, or if you start blaming yourself, the lapse may become the starting point of a relapse. Stay calm and regain control of the behavior.

Acknowledge what happened before the lapse occurred. The circumstances leading up to the lapse are more important to your progress than the negative behavior itself. In chapter 7 you discovered your own high-risk situations for overeating. These can apply to other types of lapses as well. Whether it's the people you're with, the social environment, or your emotions, these situations trigger a lapse. After the lapse, analyze the situation during which the slip occurred using the Break the Chain Activity from chapter 7. Learn something new from the lapse, so that the next time you find yourself in that situation, you're prepared to deal with it more effectively.

Review and renew your long- and short-term health goals. Are you keeping them visible? Look back over the progress you've made so far and all the weekly action steps you've accomplished. Through review and renewal, you'll get back your positive attitude about weight management and be in a better position to prevent a relapse.

Take immediate action. What you do after a lapse is just as important as understanding what brought it on. If you attack the lapse, deal with it quickly, maintain control of the situation, and move forward once again, you're treating the lapse as a minor setback and preventing it from sabotaging your weight management plan.

Getting Down to Business

Following these steps will help you prevent relapse, but they don't address the specifics—the practical ways to stay on track with weight loss and prevent lapses from feeling out of control. These come next. Provided here are Take Action Today tips that give you specific strategies for dealing with lapses and preventing them from becoming a relapse.

Take Action Today

When your motivation is low, minimize your personal high-risk situations.

Set a weight regain maximum of 2 to 3 pounds. When you hit this point, take corrective action by double-checking your portion sizes, tracking your calories to make sure you're not overeating, or adding an extra exercise session.

If you're suddenly having trouble normalizing your blood glucose levels, record all your meals for 2 days and make adjustments where needed. Another option is to plan out the next day's meals and snacks the night before.

If you're in the middle of an overeating session, start an activity that you can't do at the same time as eating, such as playing the piano or saxophone, typing, jumping rope, or knitting.

When you find yourself eating for reasons other than hunger, follow the 20-minute rule. Find an activity to do for 20 minutes, such as walking or taking a shower, that removes you from the tempting environment. After 20 minutes, the urge to eat will have passed.

After a lapse, especially one that frustrates you considerably, write in your journal about how you felt before, during, and after the situation. Just let your honest thoughts flow freely. Then write about how you will handle the situation differently the next time.

Have you ever overeaten at one meal, thrown your arms up in the air, and said, "I just blew it for the whole day. I'll start over tomorrow"? Don't let one meal throw you off course for the whole day. If you return to your normal eating habits for the remaining meals that day, you'll still be on track. Calculating the calories eaten in that one meal can help to put it into perspective, showing you that the whole day is not off course.

If your lapse is an overeating binge and you're still feeling tempted by a particular food, wait until you've regained self-control and dispose of the

---

I did it. Over the holidays, I regained all the weight I had lost. What now?

NO QUESTION IS SILLY

Analyze the situation. Did specific events throw you off track? Were you stressed out from all the additional time commitments during the holiday season? Really think through the string of lapses that led to relapse. Then review your goals. Are they still what you want to achieve? Was your original time frame realistic? Reviewing previous action steps will help you get back on track. Start with actions that motivated you the first time. This immediate action will get you back on track. But before you jump back in, be sure to develop a plan for relapse prevention so that when the next holiday season rolls around, you have your plan of attack.

food. By disposing of the food during the overeating episode, you may end up eating more.

Write each of your high-risk situations on the front of a note card. On the back of the card, write down all the ways you can deal with these situations. Then when you are in the midst of one of them, you have ready-to-use coping skills.

Although certain foods such as peanut butter or chocolate may tempt you, it's best not to avoid them completely. Learning to enjoy these craved foods in planned situations will prevent you from feeling deprived can prevent a lapse of overeating from ever occurring.

One remaining step is to identify what weekly action steps you'll incorporate into your weight management program to deal with your own lapses. Review some of your food triggers from chapter 7, consider other sabotaging health behaviors you may have, and list ways you'll manage these situations on the Lapse Management Plan work sheet (page 156). Use some of the ideas presented here or other ideas of your own.

Dealing with lapses and preventing relapse are skills you'll use throughout the entire weight and diabetes management process. In fact, these skills are probably the most crucial to achieving long-term behavior change. So even though you might be on a major success run right now, take time out to envision how you'll manage lapses when they do occur. They will happen! They're a normal part of the process. Learning to handle them effectively is the trick to staying on track with your program.

Lapse Management Plan

1. A high-risk situation for me is _____

Action steps to control this lapse and prevent relapse are _____

_____

_____

_____

_____

2. A high-risk situation for me is _____

_____

Action steps to control this lapse and prevent relapse are _____

_____

_____

_____

_____

3. A high-risk situation for me is _____

_____

Action steps to control this lapse and prevent relapse are _____

_____

_____

_____

_____

mind over matter

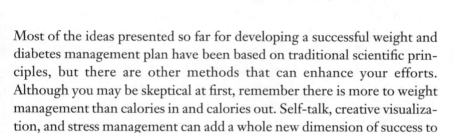

**Whether you think you can
or think you can't, you're right.**
Henry Ford

Most of the ideas presented so far for developing a successful weight and diabetes management plan have been based on traditional scientific principles, but there are other methods that can enhance your efforts. Although you may be skeptical at first, remember there is more to weight management than calories in and calories out. Self-talk, creative visualization, and stress management can add a whole new dimension of success to your journey.

Self-Talk

What emotion do you experience when a ringing phone awakens you at 2 A.M.? Most people feel fear, anticipating bad news. How about when you meet someone for the first time? You probably draw some conclusions based on his or her appearance and nonverbal communication. These are examples of how moments in life are affected by past experiences. Although you're not consciously aware of them, your mind stores all of your past encounters. The strength of your reaction to a new situation is determined by the pattern of similar past experiences, responses stored in your subconscious, and the emotions attached to them. This is why advertising slogans are so effective. "Just do it." "Baseball, hot dogs, apple pie, and Chevrolet." "It's the real thing." Each slogan evokes an emotional response to the product. You can quickly name each product because Nike, Chevrolet, and Coke have repeated their slogans to you frequently in attempts to sway your emotions so that you'll purchase their products.

The same is true of your own thoughts and ideas. You're constantly generating thoughts about yourself—your health, body size and shape, and competency in your work and relationships. These thoughts "program" your subconscious mind, establishing your attitudes and feelings about yourself. In the end, your self-image affects your actions and whether you succeed or fail in various areas of your life. For example, every time you look in the mirror, you may say to yourself, "No matter how much weight I lose, I'll never get rid of this gut!" This thought lowers your self-image and confidence, affecting your motivation to lose weight.

Although this statement was negative, the messages you send yourself can be positive. If they're positive, forgiving, and loving, you're destined for success. The problem is, since childhood you may have been trained to downplay your own abilities, skills, and talents. Because of this, you'll most likely doubt your capabilities and underestimate your self-worth as an adult. All these negative thoughts take root in your subconscious, making you uncertain about how you can keep off the lost weight or making you question whether you can maintain the day-to-day routine necessary to manage diabetes.

But you can begin to reprogram your subconscious by using a technique called self-talk. It's as simple as the name implies. By verbalizing positive messages frequently and continually, you'll retrain your mind to be motivated, energized, and on track with your weight and diabetes management plan (or any other area of your life where you'd like to make some changes).

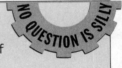

The positive self-talk in this chapter sounds very similar to the affirmations I've been using since reading about them in an earlier chapter. Are they the same? If not, how are they different?

Affirmations are really a part of self-talk. In using affirmations, you're making positive statements about yourself and your health. Self-talk is more encompassing. It's like teaching yourself a whole new internal language. You may use self-talk to confront old attitudes and beliefs, combat negative mental images and programming, or improve your self-image. Whereas affirmations are a process of repeating positive messages, self-talk is an inner dialogue with your subconscious. If you've found success with affirmations, continue to use them and consider expanding your positive messages to include self-talk.

To get started on improving your self-talk, listen to the messages you currently send yourself. Every time you make a negative statement or have a negative thought about yourself, write it down on the Talk Back With Self-Talk work sheet (page 160). Do this for 1 to 2 weeks. Negative self-talk can be subtle, so listen closely to the messages. Some examples of negative messages are

"I can't do it."

"I'm going to be late for work again."

"Why should I try, it probably won't work anyway."

"I'm always going to have a weight problem."

"I know he or she won't like me."

"I'm just not good at athletics."

Once you have a list of negative self-talk messages, categorize them. Do most relate to your body size and shape? Your health? Your job performance? Categorizing the messages will give you an idea of where to start. You may choose to work on negative health and body messages, considering your current focus on health management, even though they're not highest in number. As you've been doing with weekly action steps, it's best to work on just one area of self-talk at a time.

Next, review the chosen category of negative messages and write some positive statements to counter them. Again, use the Talk Back With Self-Talk work sheet provided. Make your positive statements simple, clear, and consistent with the health goals you've set. Examples of positive self-talk to combat negative messages mentioned earlier are

Negative: Why should I try? It probably won't work anyway.
Positive: I will try and acknowledge that I may have to try several times before I succeed.

Negative: I'm always going to have a weight problem.
Positive: Today is the first day of the rest of my life. I can manage my weight by taking one day at a time.

Negative: I know he or she won't like me.
Positive: I have many likable characteristics and traits. People will enjoy meeting and getting to know me.

You can write your positive self-talk messages on the work sheet, but it's best to keep them with you throughout the day as a reminder. Write them on note cards, post them on your bathroom mirror or computer screen, or

Talk Back With Self-Talk

1. Negative messages I send myself: _____

I can't resist dessert when eating out. (7) _____

_____

_____

_____

_____

_____

_____

_____

_____

_____

_____

2. Categories of my negative self-talk? (check all that apply)
   - ❏ 1. body size and shape
   - ❏ 2. interpersonal relationships
   - ❏ 3. work performance
   - ❏ 4. physical activity
   - ❏ 5. intelligence
   - ❏ 6. diabetes management
   - ❏ 7. self-control
   - ❏ 8. other:

3. By using the numbers indicated in step 2, assign each statement in step 1 a category (see example).

4. Category of negative messages to work on: _____

5. Positive self-talk I will use to combat negative messages: _____

_____

_____

_____

_____

_____

record them on a cassette tape that you can play back several times during the day.

When you first start practicing the art of self-talk, you'll notice some internal arguments between your old and new programming. To win the argument, repeat your positive messages frequently. Remember that saying them out loud is most effective, because another sense—your hearing—becomes involved in the process. It may take several weeks for the positive self-talk to take over, but the results will be worth the effort.

Visualize Success

Creative visualization is similar in many ways to self-talk, except visualization uses images rather than verbal statements to combat negative thoughts. Professional athletes use imagery to maximize their performance. Actors use it to get inside a role. If you tend to learn better through visual means, this may be just what you need to change habits.

To begin using creative visualization, find a quiet spot where you can relax. Using one of the negative messages from step 1 of the Talk Back With Self-Talk work sheet, follow these three steps:

1. Set an action step. One example is "I will no longer get queasy when doing finger pricks to check my blood sugars."

2. Create a picture in your mind of how you'd like the situation to be. For example, if you get nervous as the clock ticks closer to the scheduled time for checking your blood glucose levels, create an image of yourself doing the task. Are you sitting or standing when you do the finger prick? Where are you? In what room of your house? Which finger are you using? Imagine your opposite hand as steady and your mood as calm and relaxed. Visualize how quickly the stick is done and the abundant drop of blood that results. Did you really feel any pain at all? Run the test. Read the results. What action do you need to take? Picture yourself with a matter-of-fact attitude about the whole process. Notice how not more than a minute or two has passed; the whole process was so quick and easy. Keep your image in the present, not the future.

3. Focus on this picture often. Once you have the image detailed, commit it to memory. Then every chance you get, think of it. In quiet moments before you fall asleep at night, during your morning shower, while you exercise, and as frequently as you can throughout the day, replay this image.

Be patient with creative visualization. The new image may take some time to take root, but you'll begin to notice a change in your comfort level with pricking your finger and in your attitudes about how you control your diabetes.

Stress Management

You can use self-talk and creative visualization to improve control of your stress level, but there are other techniques yet to come. Keep in mind, though, that the goal is not to eliminate all stress from your life. Some stress is good; it keeps you motivated, challenged, and satisfied. Life would be boring without it. As in many areas of health, however, moderation is the key. Too much stress is damaging to your health. Muscle tension, headaches, and stomach problems are common symptoms. Chronic stress can lead to serious health problems such as heart disease, increased blood glucose levels, and other complications with diabetes. Not only your physical well-being but also your mental health, relationships, and work performance are affected.

For success in weight and diabetes management, the goal is to minimize and manage the factors that add stress to your life. Begin by identifying where the tension comes from. In general there are four main categories of stressors:

Environmental—pollution, traffic, noise, weather

Social—marriage or divorce, finances, job strain, death of a parent or child

Physiological—sleep disorders, aging, menopause, living with a chronic disease

Internal—perfectionism, self-esteem issues, personality traits

The tricky thing is that stress factors are very individual. While you feel overwhelmed by last-minute deadlines, your coworker thrives in this environment. By the same token, the announcement that your parents are getting divorced doesn't affect you as much as it does your sibling. To learn what stresses you out, use the Stress Monitor work sheet on the following page.

Although there's no exact score that says you have too much or too little stress, the object of this work sheet is to determine if the majority of your stress is coming from one area or if it's split across the categories.

Stress Monitor

Check any of the following experiences that you've had within the past year or that you expect to happen within the next year.

Environmental Factors

❑ Pollution

❑ Excessive noise

❑ Weather extremes

❑ Frequent travel

❑ Limited sunlight exposure

❑ Difficult commute

Social Factors

❑ Marriage or divorce

❑ Death of a loved one

❑ Birth or adoption of baby

❑ Major purchase (home, etc.)

❑ Job change

❑ Frequent conflicts with family members, coworkers, or friends

❑ Financial problems

❑ Too many family or household responsibilities

Physiological Factors

❑ Lack of sleep

❑ Physical disability

❑ Chronic disease

❑ Excessive drinking

❑ Aging

❑ Menopause

❑ Smoking

❑ Sleep disorder

❑ Physical injury

Internal Factors

❑ Perfectionism

❑ Chronic worry

❑ Unrealistic expectations (of self or others)

❑ Overreacting

❑ All-or-nothing thinking

Total Number of Stressors

_____ Environmental   _____ Social

_____ Physiological   _____ Internal

_____ GRAND TOTAL

Identifying the stressors in your life is the first step toward minimizing them.

Use the following ideas to learn to cope with your tensions and manage your personal stressors. As always, consider these tips for upcoming weekly action steps.

Take Action Today

Keep a time log. Poor time management can contribute to stress. To improve your time management skills, keep a log of how you're spending your time. Log your entries in 1/4-, 1/2-, or 1-hour time blocks. Logging your actions for a week or two helps you realize when time is wasted in your day and where you can simplify actions and steps. Additionally, you'll have a better handle on how long tasks and projects actually take, so that you can plan more appropriately in the future.

Change how you react to situations. Although circumstances and people may not change, you always have the option of changing your reaction to them.

Get a massage. Whether from a professional massage therapist, family member, or friend, even a 5-minute back or shoulder rub can relieve tension and stress, helping you to relax.

Exercise. Not only does exercise provide an immediate stress break, but it also releases endorphins into your bloodstream, which lighten your mood.

Learn to delegate. Although others might not do it exactly like you, consider what tasks you can delegate to kids, partner, roommate, or coworker.

Separate work and home. You may leave one set of stressors at the office only to be met with varied family and household responsibilities when you walk in the door. Between work and home, find 15 to 20 minutes to mentally and emotionally transition to the new environment.

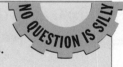

My boss creates major stress in my life. He's constantly hounding me, giving me projects that he doesn't have time for, and then expecting me to meet short deadlines. What can I say to get him to quit stressing me out?

When a particular situation or environment causes you a significant amount of tension, it's not uncommon to blame the other person or situation and take no responsibility yourself. But consider your circle of influence. Complete the statement "I can make the situation better by . . ." Try finding a stress reliever such as a racquetball game or walk over the lunch hour. Work with the people involved to determine which time lines can be pushed back. Changing how you react and handle the situation that is causing you stress is within your power.

Write "to do" lists. At the start of your day, make a list of everything you hope to accomplish that day. Prioritize the tasks. Then cross off the lowest priority items on the list and move ahead with a realistic plan for the day.

Identify stressors. Brainstorm a list of situations that cause you stress. Arrange the list from least stressful to most stressful. Create a list of personal coping strategies for the five most stressful situations on your list.

Learn to say no. Before agreeing to take on a project, ask yourself how you feel about the request being made. Do you really want to do it? Make sure you know what you're being asked to do. Say no without feeling guilty or making excuses if it's something you're really not interested in doing or if you can't commit yourself to the time and work involved.

Laugh. A big belly laugh that brings you close to tears completely relaxes your body, distracts you from the stressor, and sheds new light on the situation.

Stretch during your work day. Take a few minutes for shoulder rolls, toe touches, and side bends to relax your muscles and give your mind a refreshing break.

Sleep. Find the amount of sleep you need to be at your best and get it every night.

Your Mind: A Powerful Tool

Open your mind to a new way of thinking. You may not even realize the impact your thoughts, attitudes, and stress level have on your actions and habits. Mind over matter can be a powerful tool in your lifestyle "fix-up" project. Once you try these techniques, you'll see that they have helped you move one step closer to success in weight and diabetes management.

a lifetime of health

Desire it, choose it, act it, and keep on keeping on.
Earnie Larsen

AN ACTION PLAN

You read and hear statistics all the time about the number of people who've lost weight, only to gain it back within 5 years. It's true that maintaining a lower weight is often more difficult than losing the weight in the first place. But this doesn't mean it can't be done. Countless other statistics detail the individuals who've lost weight and kept it off for more than 20 years. It's within your reach to be in the second group of statistics, to be a lifetime maintainer.

As you now know, losing weight in order to improve diabetes control involves more than balancing the calories you eat with the calories you burn in daily activity and exercise. Stress management, a solid support network, treating lapses as minor setbacks, and a variety of other skills affect your success in losing weight, controlling diabetes, and building new health habits. The same is true of maintaining the lost weight and new behaviors. The goal of this chapter is to help you transition to this next phase, the maintenance phase of weight and diabetes management.

Transition Time

You've learned a lot about what it takes to lose weight and manage diabetes. But what does it take to maintain a weight loss? Although the new habits you've built need to be continued, there are definitely areas where you can relax your guidelines. Doing this can be scary, though, because there's always the potential that you'll regain the weight or completely slip back into your old habits. Also, you don't want to jeopardize the improved control of diabetes you've achieved. So you need to find the right mix of new habits and a comfort level with your healthier lifestyle. As you strive to find this balance, there are six attributes that will help you successfully transition to maintaining your new lifestyle habits.

Personal Responsibility. Stop right now and give yourself a pat on the back and smile in the mirror to acknowledge the success you've had in improving your lifestyle and taking charge of your diabetes, weight, and health. No matter what that number is on the scale, you deserve to recognize all you've done to make it this far. Most people seldom stop and reflect on the positive changes they've made, the hard work done, or the progress made toward their goals. It deserves to be savored. Take the rest of the day to feel positively fabulous about your success.

Acknowledging your success is one part of personal responsibility, but the other key is realizing that no one but you can keep the weight off. You're the only one who could make yourself lose weight—no matter what your health care provider, spouse, or friends said. From deep inside yourself, you found the motivation and energy to change your lifestyle. The same is required in long-term weight and diabetes management. It's up to you, and nobody but you, to maintain your new health behaviors.

Consistency. People who've lost significant amounts of weight often fall back into their old habits without even realizing what they're doing. They rationalize that skipping exercise one day or eating an extra portion of french fries won't hurt. But soon it's a month of days without exercise or it's eating "traditional" treats such as ice cream or potato chips every night. It's true that shifting to weight maintenance means you can be less strict with your habits, but you still need to be consistent with the positive health changes you've made.

In the long run, it's better to exercise 1 day a week for a year than 3 days a week for 2 months. You'll have better long-term management of your weight and diabetes if you lower your fat grams to a level you can follow indefinitely rather than eating no fat for 3 months just to lose weight. When transitioning to weight maintenance, you may be able to miss an occasional support group session or, on rare occasion, react to your emotions by eating too much, but in general you want to continue with the new, healthier lifestyle you've built. The habits you formed during weight loss will help you maintain your weight loss for a lifetime.

Balance and Moderation. It's important to be conscientious about habits that might cause your weight to fluctuate, but this doesn't mean you can't ever eat pie or candy or spend an evening as a couch potato. Practice the 80/20 rule. Balance and moderation mean that if 80 percent of the time you make really healthy food and lifestyle choices, the other 20 percent can fall through the cracks without your health being adversely affected. Holidays, vacations, and special occasions fall into the 20 percent category. Consider choosing this rule as your motto for weight maintenance and diabetes control.

Empowerment. You couldn't have examined and changed behaviors or created a healthier you without a sense of empowerment. This attitude is essential as you move into maintenance. Empowerment means taking responsibility for your own life and, in this case, your own health. It means taking time away from other things, and sometimes other people, to exercise, attend a support group, or relax in a calming environment. Others may assume that because you've lost the weight you wanted to lose, you don't need to bother with all the "stuff" you were taking time out for anymore. Be firm in your resolution to continually make time for your health.

Action Oriented. Action steps were a valuable tool for gradually replacing old habits with healthier ones. Just because you've lost the weight doesn't mean you're through with action steps. Although the focus may change, there are still habits and behaviors you need continually to work on as a part of maintenance, and the best way to do this is with small, gradual changes each week.

I'm still having trouble keeping weight off. Any advice?

NO QUESTION IS SILLY

One way to handle this is initially to lose only 1/3 of your total weight goal. Once you've achieved this weight loss, work on maintaining this new weight—not losing more weight—for 2 to 3 months. Doing this will give you confidence and help you build the habits you need to maintain a lower weight.

When you're comfortable at this lower weight, return to your weight loss mode. Again, aim for 1/3 of your goal, and once there, maintain this newer weight for 2 to 3 months. Continue this process until you reach your overall goal.

Although it may take longer to lose weight this way, in the end you'll not only be healthier but have learned how to maintain a weight loss.

Self-Monitoring. People who are successful at long-term weight maintenance develop a monitoring system. Some examples include tracking fat
grams a few days a week, setting an upper weight limit that, when reached,
signals that positive habits need to be tightened up, or establishing a personal range within which to consistently keep your blood glucose level.
Decide on a self-monitoring system that will help you prevent small lapses
that could add up to a relapse.

Watching Yourself

Probably the most important component of weight maintenance is your
self-monitoring system. You lived with your old habits for most of your life
and have only recently made changes for a healthier lifestyle. You'll have
to make a conscious effort to prevent falling back into your old habits and
losing all the progress you've made.

Your self-monitoring system should be as individualized as your weight
loss and diabetes management plan. Consider your lifestyle, habits, family
situation, and personality when designing a method for monitoring your
maintenance. The following three work sheets will help.

1. Tools for Success (next page) walks you through steps to identify the five
skills most important to your individualized weight maintenance program.

2. High-Risk Solutions (page 172) encourages you to anticipate situations
that put you in jeopardy of losing control of your health habits and to plan
how you'll confront them. By thinking this through ahead of time, you'll
be prepared when any of the situations actually occur. Review your food
triggers from chapter 7 and high-risk situations identified in chapter 13,
because some of these issues will affect you as you move into the maintenance phase.

3. Progress Reports (page 173) provides space for you to chart your continued progress in weight and diabetes management. Although your focus has
been on weekly action steps, periodic check-ins on your long- and short-
term goals are important. Review the health goals you set in chapter 6, and
as you move forward on the time line, chart your accomplishments here.

Tools for Success

1. Collect supplies for this activity: writing utensil and stopwatch or timer.

2. For the next 3 minutes, quickly write down skills you've gained during the weight loss phase of your weight management plan. (Examples: limiting portion sizes, exercising three times a week, finding alternative outlets for emotional upsets.)

_____

_____

_____

_____

_____

_____

_____

_____

3. Review the list and rank the five that are most important to your success in weight maintenance.

_____

_____

_____

_____

_____

_____

_____

_____

4. Keep your Top Five Skills list visible and refer to it often.

High-Risk Solutions

1. List situations, environments, or people that jeopardize the healthy habits you have built.

_____

_____

_____

_____

_____

_____

2. List events or life changes you anticipate during the next 3 months that may affect your ability to maintain your new habits. (Examples: holidays, vacations, child's wedding, job change.)

_____

_____

_____

_____

_____

3. Brainstorm methods you will use to confront these high-risk situations. (examples: find support group, schedule exercise as if it were a business meeting, attend only my favorite holiday parties.)

_____

_____

_____

_____

_____

Progress Reports

Weight maintenance goal: _____

Time line _____

Achieved? _____

Actions taken: _____

_____

_____

Success story to tell: _____

_____

_____

_____

_____

_____

Weight maintenance goal: _____

Time line _____

Achieved? _____

Actions taken: _____

_____

_____

Success story to tell: _____

_____

_____

_____

_____

_____

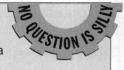

The other day I browsed through a bookstore and was overwhelmed by the number of health books. I left without buying a thing because I didn't know how to make a good choice. Any advice?

Although there are an unbelievable number of health resources available, it's possible to make some smart choices that will be useful for you. The most important step is determining if the author is credible. Whether for a book, cookbook, newsletter, magazine article, video or cassette tape, or Internet site, assess potential resources using the following criteria:

Who wrote the publication? The initials RD indicate the person is a registered dietitian. With extensive training and national accreditation, RDs are truly nutrition experts. LNs (licensed nutritionists) and LDs (licensed dietitians) have similar backgrounds. The initials CDE stand for certified diabetes educator and indicate the person has expertise in the area of diabetes. Medical doctors (MD) and registered nurses (RN) are other professionals you can trust as authors, but you should consider the type of book they're writing. Neither of these professionals has nutrition training, but for resources on diabetes care and medical issues related to diabetes, they would be credible authors. Be wary of the use of PhD. Although individuals with these credentials can call themselves doctor (Dr.), they're not necessarily medical doctors, and their PhD isn't always in a health field.

Are the promises believable? Any publication that guarantees you'll lose 5 pounds in a week or 10 inches in a month is simply trying to take your money.

Are sound principles taught? The cabbage diet, the steam room technique for weight loss—titles such as these appear frequently on magazine covers. Don't be fooled. Health resources that recommend you eat foods in a certain order, instruct you to eat only one food for days, or suggest that honey isn't really sugar should be left on the bookstore shelf.

Using these criteria may help you narrow the list of potential resources, but there will still be a lot to choose from. Consider checking out some titles at your local library to see if you really want to spend the money to purchase them. Ask your health care team what additional resources they recommend. Or at a support group meeting for persons with diabetes, find out what others with your health condition are using as additional resources.

Motivating Yourself for Maintenance

The previous work sheets will help you maintain the new health habits you've built, but as you move into a lifetime of maintenance, you'll periodically find your motivation waning. You might get bored with walking on your treadmill or the same old healthy lunches. This tendency, sometimes called "wandering," is OK as long as you find a way to get back on track. The following tips give ideas on how to stay motivated and energized during this lifelong phase of weight management.

Try a new form of exercise each year. In-line skating, aerobic boxing, and step aerobics may be the latest craze, but something different that might intrigue you is on the horizon. What about rock climbing or kayaking for a totally new activity experience?

Form your own support group. Most likely, there are people in your worksite or neighborhood who are managing weight or health problems, too. As a group, meet weekly or monthly to discuss issues you each face and support one another in your efforts. By finding people in close proximity, you'll be more likely to stick with this support group.

Start a "healthy gourmet" dinner club. Find others who are interested in trying exotic or not so exotic cuisine that's been modified with health in mind. Meet once a month or every other month and enjoy the new tastes and the company.

Find opportunities to refresh your attitude. Look to community education or the local university for classes or conferences with themes of motivation or personal renewal. Everyone needs a pick-me-up now and again.

Make your exercise routines more interesting. Pick a place on the map that you've always wanted to visit—the Florida Keys, San Francisco, or Australia. Calculate the miles from your home to the destination. On a map, log your weekly miles (walked, ran, or biked) to your vacation. Set a goal date of when you plan to reach the site. Once you achieve your goal, reward yourself with plane tickets to the destination or some memento of the locale (such as San Francisco sourdough bread).

Keep a health journal. Make note of blood lipid (cholesterol, HDL, LDL, triglyceride) values, body fat measurements, hemoglobin A1c levels, or any other health parameter. After a year, make a chart or graph of the changes you've made happen in these numbers. Success itself can be a great motivator, especially when it's visual. You'll be able to see how all those little action steps have added up to big changes.

Take a vacation that caters to the health-conscious. Many cruises offer this option. Biking from inn to inn is popular in the Northeast. White-water rafting trips are offered on many rivers in the United States.

Sign up for a "fun run," "walk for a cause," minitriathalon, or similar event in your local community. Set a goal just to finish the event or a personal time you hope to accomplish.

Hire a personal trainer. Sometimes all you need is someone to push you that extra step or show you a new exercise routine. Because exercise is their profession, personal trainers are up-to-date on the latest tricks of their trade and may be just what you need for a boost of energy.

Volunteer with a local health organization such as the American Diabetes Association or American Heart Association. The many benefits to you include meeting other people interested in improving their health, getting a visual reminder of why you need to continue your efforts for a healthy lifestyle, and perhaps motivating someone else with the success you've had in building new habits.

The Final Act

Think back to the ladder of diabetes care detailed in chapter 1. The rungs of the ladder were

diabetes care
stress management
support
monitoring
physical activity
meal planning

As the ladder shows, control of diabetes, weight management, and overall good health are all intertwined. The actions you've taken and new habits you've built as you moved from rung to rung create positive results in all three areas. The climb to the top of your own health ladder has put you in charge of your lifestyle, made you feel positive about your diabetes care and weight, and given you energy for the future. In the beginning you may have felt overwhelmed by your diabetes diagnosis, but now you have the skills, knowledge, and motivation to move forward with a life in which diabetes is a minor inconvenience instead of a debilitating disease.

Appendix A
Fat and Calorie Counts

FOOD	AMOUNT	CALORIES	FAT GRAMS
Breads and grains			
bagel, plain or water	1 (3 1/2")	195	2
biscuit, baking powder	1 (2")	100	5
bread	1 slice	80	1
cereal, most types	3/4 cup	80	2
granola	1/4 cup	120	5
crackers			
graham	2 (2 1/2" square)	60	1
oyster	10	33	1
saltines	6	78	1
croissant	1 (2 oz.)	234	12
egg noodles, cooked	1 cup	212	2
English muffin	1	154	1
muffin	1 medium	216	7
noodles or pasta	1 cup	197	1
oatmeal, cooked	1 cup	145	2
pancake	1 (4" diameter)	83	3
rice, white, cooked	1 cup	162	0
roll (hamburger or hot dog)	1	114	2
tortilla, corn	1 (6")	60	1
flour	1 (6")	81	2
waffle, frozen	1	103	4

FOOD	AMOUNT	CALORIES	FAT GRAMS
Combination foods			
beef and vegetable stir-fry	1 1/2 cups	285	9
beef stew with vegetables	1 cup	220	11
chili with beans	1 cup	286	14
chow mein, beef, pork, chicken	1 cup	255	10
egg roll, frozen	1 large	150	6
fettucini Alfredo	1 cup	380	20
frozen low-calorie entrée	1 (8 oz.)	220	7
Hamburger Helper	1 cup	280	8
lasagna, meat	4" × 4"	240	8
macaroni and cheese	1 cup	320	12
pot pie, frozen	1	435	25
Salisbury steak with gravy	11 oz.	525	32
spaghetti with meatballs	1 cup	300	11
with meat sauce	1 cup	265	15
with tomato sauce	1 cup	190	9
soup, chicken noodle	1 cup	75	7
cream of mushroom	1 cup	200	14
black bean	1 cup	115	2
tuna noodle casserole	1 cup	240	7
tuna salad, regular	1/2 cup	190	10
veal parmigiana, cutlet	4 oz.	240	12
Desserts and snacks			
apple pie	1/8 pie	282	12
candy corn	14 pieces	182	1
caramels	9 pieces	271	6
carbonated beverages	12-oz. can	151	0
chips, baked tortilla	1 oz. (20 chips)	110	1
chips, corn	1 oz.	153	9
potato	1 oz.	150	10
tortilla	1 oz.	150	8
cake, angel food	1/12 cake	126	0
cake doughnut	1	105	6
chocolate chip cookie	1 small (2" cookie)	50	3
chocolate-flavored syrup (thin type)	2 tbsp.	82	0
fig bar	1	60	1
gingerbread, from 8" square cake	1/9 cake	174	4
gingersnaps, vanilla wafers	2	60	1
gumdrops	10 small	135	0

FOOD	AMOUNT	CALORIES	FAT GRAMS
ice cream, regular, vanilla	1/2 cup	132	7
soft serve	1/2 cup	111	3
jam, jelly preserves	1 tbsp.	50	0
jelly beans	10 large	104	0
licorice	1 oz.	100	0
marshmallows	1 oz.	90	0
milk chocolate	1 oz.	150	9
popcorn, air popped	3 cups	90	1
oil popped	3 cups	123	6
pound cake (1/17 of loaf)	1-oz. slice	142	9
sandwich-type cookies (1 3/4")	2	100	4
sherbet	1/2 cup	130	2
sugar, brown, powdered, white	1 tbsp.	52	0
syrup, maple	1 tbsp.	52	0
yogurt, frozen, soft serve	8 oz.	140	4
Eggs			
eggs (whole), large	1	75	5
egg white	1	17	0
Fats and oils			
butter or margarine	1 tbsp.	100	12
reduced-calorie margarine	1 tbsp.	50	6
oil (any type)	1 tbsp.	120	14
shortening	1 tbsp.	110	13
salad dressing (regular)	1 tbsp.	68	7
mayonnaise	1 tbsp.	100	12
reduced fat	1 tbsp.	50	5
cream cheese	2 tbsp.	100	10
Fish, poultry, meat			
fish (skinless, flesh only, cooked without added fat or sauces)			
white-fleshed fish	3 oz.	100	2
catfish	3 oz.	130	7
mackerel, Atlantic, Pacific	3 oz.	171	9
rainbow trout	3 oz.	144	6
salmon, Atlantic, coho	3 oz.	154	7
oysters	12 medium	116	4
shrimp and other shellfish	3 oz.	85	1
chicken (roasted, meat only, no skin)			
breast	3 oz.	140	3
leg	3 oz.	163	7
thigh	3 oz.	178	9

FOOD	AMOUNT	CALORIES	FAT GRAMS
turkey (cooked, meat only, no skin)			
breast	3 oz.	121	2
dark meat	3 oz.	160	6
ground (broiled)	3 oz.	200	11
lean beef (cooked, meat only, trimmed of fat)			
eye of round	3 oz.	138	4
top round	3 oz	163	6
top sirloin	3 oz.	176	7
tenderloin	3 oz.	117	5
flank	3 oz.	192	9
ground, 85% lean	3 oz.	225	13
ground, 80% lean	3 oz.	248	16
lean pork (cooked, meat only, trimmed of fat)			
tenderloin	3 oz.	141	4
chop (sirloin, loin, rib)	3 oz.	119	7
boneless loin roast	3 oz.	142	6
boneless rib roast	3 oz.	160	9
processed lunch meats			
bologna, beef	1 oz.	88	8
chicken or turkey breast	1 oz.	33	1
Canadian bacon	1 oz.	52	2
ham	1 oz.	52	3
summer sausage	1 oz.	95	8
turkey ham	1 oz.	36	1

Fruits and vegetables

FOOD	AMOUNT	CALORIES	FAT GRAMS
avocado	1/8	38	4
baked potato	1 medium	220	0
coconut, dried, sweetened, flaked	1/4 cup	117	8
french fries, deep fried	10	158	8
frozen, oven baked	10	125	4
fruit, fresh, canned, or juice	1/2 cup	60	0
potato salad (made with mayonnaise)	1/2 cup	180	11
scalloped potatoes (homemade)	1/2 cup	105	5
vegetables, fresh, canned, or frozen	1/2 cup	30	0

Milk products

FOOD	AMOUNT	CALORIES	FAT GRAMS
cheese			
American, blue, cheddar, Swiss	1 oz.	100	9
feta	1 oz.	75	6
mozzarella, part skim	1 oz.	81	5
Parmesan cheese, grated	1 tbsp.	29	2
cottage cheese			
1% fat	1/2 cup	92	1
2% fat	1/2 cup	101	2
4% fat	1/2 cup	109	5

FOOD	AMOUNT	CALORIES	FAT GRAMS
milk			
skim	1 cup	86	0
low fat	1 cup	102	3
reduced fat	1 cup	121	5
whole	1 cup	150	8
yogurt (made with low-fat milk)			
fruit flavored	8 oz.	190	3
plain	8 oz.	140	4
Nuts and legumes			
beans			
baked	1/4 cup	65	1
garbanzo, kidney, pinto	1/4 cup	60	1
refried, fat free	1/4 cup	68	0
nuts			
almonds	1 oz.	167	15
cashews	1 oz.	163	14
peanuts	1 oz. (1/4 cup)	170	14
pecans	1 oz.	190	19
walnuts	1 oz.	182	18
peanut butter, regular	1 tbsp.	94	8
reduced fat	1 tbsp.	95	6
tofu, soybean curd	1/2 cup	94	6

Restaurants, fast food

Arby's

Junior Roast Beef	1	233	11
Regular Roast Beef	1	383	18
French Dip	1	368	15
Ham 'n Cheese	1	355	14
Light Roast Beef Deluxe	1	294	10
Light Roast Turkey Deluxe	1	260	6
Light Roast Chicken Deluxe	1	276	7
Garden Salad	1	117	5
Chef Salad	1	205	10

Burger King

Whopper	1	630	38
Whopper With Cheese	1	720	46
Cheeseburger	1	300	14
Jr. Whopper With Cheese	1	380	22
Hamburger	1	260	10
BK Big Fish Sandwich	1	710	43

FOOD	AMOUNT	CALORIES	FAT GRAMS
Chicken Tenders	6 piece	236	13
Chunky Chicken Salad	1	142	4
Garden Salad	1	95	5
French Fries	medium	372	20
Vanilla Shake	medium	310	6
Dairy Queen			
Single Hamburger	1	290	12
Single Hamburger With Cheese	1	340	17
Hot Dog	1	240	14
Hot Dog With Chili	1	280	16
BBQ Beef Sandwich	1	225	4
Grilled Chicken Sandwich	1	310	10
French Fries	regular	300	14
Cone	regular	340	10
Chocolate Sundae	small	300	7
Vanilla Malt	small	610	14
Banana Split	1	510	11
Buster Bar	1	450	29
Dilly Bar	1	210	13
Heath Blizzard	small	560	23
Strawberry Breeze	small	290	0
Domino's Pizza			
Cheese	2 slices of 12"	344	10
Pepperoni	2 slices of 12"	406	15
Sausage or Mushroom	2 slices of 12"	402	14
Veggie	2 slices of 12"	360	10
Hardee's			
Hamburger	1	260	9
Cheeseburger	1	300	13
Quarter-Pound Cheeseburger	1	490	25
Bacon Cheeseburger	1	600	36
Regular Roast Beef	1	370	16
Garden Salad	1	190	14
Chef Salad	1	200	13
Fried Chicken Breast	1	370	15
Fried Chicken Wing	1	200	13
Fried Chicken Thigh	1	330	15

FOOD	AMOUNT	CALORIES	FAT GRAMS
Cole Slaw	4 oz.	240	20
Mashed Potatoes	4 oz.	70	0
Gravy	1.5 oz.	20	0
French Fries	medium	350	15
Ham 'n Egg Biscuit	1	370	19
Biscuit 'n Gravy	1	440	24
Pancakes	3	280	2
Kentucky Fried Chicken			
Original Recipe Chicken Wing	1	150	8
Original Recipe Chicken Breast	1	360	20
Original Recipe Chicken Drumstick	1	130	7
Original Recipe Chicken Thigh	1	260	17
Chicken Sandwich	1	482	27
Hot Wings	6	471	33
Kentucky Nuggets	6	284	18
Potato Wedges	1 order	192	9
Cornbread	1 piece	175	6
Buttermilk Biscuit	1	200	12
Mashed Potatoes With Gravy	1 serving	109	5
BBB Baked Beans	1 serving	132	2
Coleslaw	1 serving	114	6
McDonald"s			
Hamburger	1	270	9
Cheeseburger	1	320	13
Quarter Pounder With Cheese	1	520	29
Big Mac	1	510	26
Filet-o-Fish	1	360	16
Chicken McNuggets	6 piece	300	18
Chicken Fajita	1	190	8
French Fries	medium	320	17
Chef Salad	1	210	11
Chunky Chicken Salad	1	160	5
Garden Salad	1	80	4
Vanilla Reduced-Fat Ice Cream Cone	1	150	5
Apple Bran Muffin	1	180	0
Egg McMuffin	1	280	11
Apple Danish	1	390	18

FOOD	AMOUNT	CALORIES	FAT GRAMS
Hot Cakes, plain	1 serving	245	4
English Muffin	1	170	4
Pizza Hut			
Pan Pizza, cheese	2 slices, medium	522	22
Pan Pizza, pepperoni	2 slices, medium	530	24
Pan Pizza, supreme	2 slices, medium	622	30
Thin 'n Crispy, cheese	2 slices, medium	410	16
Thin 'n Crispy, pepperoni	2 slices, medium	430	20
Thin 'n Crispy, supreme	2 slices, medium	514	26
Hand-Tossed, cheese	2 slices, medium	470	14
Hand-Tossed, pepperoni	2 slices, medium	476	16
Hand-Tossed, supreme	2 slices, medium	568	24
Subway			
Cold Cut Combo Sub	6"	427	20
Subway Club Sub	6"	361	12
Tuna Fish Sub	6"	551	36
Turkey Breast Sub	6"	322	10
Roast Beef Sub	6"	345	12
Ham and Cheese Sub	6"	322	9
Veggies and Cheese Sub	6"	268	9
Taco Bell			
Taco	1	180	11
Taco Supreme	1	230	15
Soft Taco	1	220	11
Chicken Soft Taco	1	213	10
Tostada	1	243	11
Bean Burrito	1	390	12
Burrito Supreme	1	440	19
Chicken Burrito	1	334	12
Nachos	1 serving	346	18
Chicken MexiMelt	1	257	15
Mexican Pizza	1	575	37
Taco Salad With Shell	1	860	55
Wendy's			
Plain Single	1	360	16
Single With Everything	1	420	20
Big Bacon Classic	1	610	33

FOOD	AMOUNT	CALORIES	FAT GRAMS
Jr. Hamburger	1	270	10
Jr. Cheeseburger	1	320	13
Grilled Chicken Sandwich	1	290	7
Chicken Club Sandwich	1	500	23
French Fries	medium	380	19
Chili	small	210	7
Plain Baked Potato	1	310	0
Bacon and Cheese Baked Potato	1	540	18
Sour Cream and Chives Baked Potato	1	380	6
Frosty	small (12 oz.)	340	10

Data Source: Nutritionist IV, version 3.0, N2 Computing. *Fast Food Facts* by the Minnesota Attorney General's Office.

Appendix B
The Enlightened
Shopping Tour

Hunting down nutritious products in the grocery store can seem like a maze with no road map provided. This tour through the supermarket will help you avoid detours and stay on track to make healthful choices.

Guiding Principles

Keep the following guiding principles in mind next time you grab the car keys and checkbook and head out the door for the store.

Shop with a list. The first stop in healthful shopping begins before you even enter the supermarket. Although it may sound like a tedious waste of time, writing a list decreases the likelihood you'll make impulsive (and maybe not the healthiest) purchases. A shopping list also encourages you to plan meals in advance and provides an opportunity to check your shelves to see what you do or don't need to stock up on.

Low fat is where it's at. As you wander the aisles, remember that your primary nutrition goal is to lower the fat in the foods you eat. Read food labels and compare the fat content of different products.

There is no substitute for taste. It's true that your goal is to shop for healthier foods. But you still want to be able to enjoy what you eat. Healthful shopping means finding the balance of good nutrition and taste that suits you. If you don't like the fat-free sour cream, but find the low-fat version just as good as regular, you've found your balance between taste and nutrition.

Strive for five. People who eat more fruits and vegetables are less likely to get cancer or heart disease. Plan for 5 servings of fruits and vegetables daily for each member of your household. Remember, it's 5 servings, not five separate fruits and/or vegetables. Choose from fresh, dried, frozen, and canned when adding up your numbers.

Whereas these are general guidelines to keep in mind when grocery shopping, the following tips will help you make nutritious choices in each section of the grocery store. The sections of the store are broken down into three categories: buying fresh, frozen, and packaged foods.

Buying Fresh

Produce

Load up your cart in this section of the store. Virtually all fruits and vegetables are fat free (avocados, olives, and coconuts are the exceptions) and high in carbohydrates. To get the full range of vitamins and minerals your body needs, choose a variety of colors from the produce area.

Buy cleaned and chopped salads, cauliflower, broccoli, pineapple, and cantaloupe if convenience is the name of your game. Try the in-store salad bar for a plan-ahead lunch or for ingredients for a stir-fry.

Fresh herbs are now commonplace in the produce section. Cilantro, parsley, oregano, and a wide variety of peppers can add flavor to any meal.

The Deli

Meats such as turkey, ham, and roast beef can be lean. They can, however, also be high in sodium.

Dressings and sauces used on salads are typically the high-fat version. Anything that is "reduced fat" is often highlighted. Choose oil-based salads such as three-bean or pasta salads topped with vinaigrette instead of creamy salads such as potato, tuna, or seafood.

Many delis provide nutrition information on their offerings. If it isn't placed in an obvious spot, ask.

Meats

Choose lean cuts of meat with the fat trimmed. Top round, top loin, eye of round, sirloin, and flank steak are lean cuts of beef. Pork cuts to consider include loin chops and roasts, tenderloin, Canadian bacon, and ham (check the sodium content on ham and Canadian bacon). Most cuts of lamb are lean, except for the shoulder. Ground veal is the only high-fat choice in this category.

Purchase skinless poultry. White meat tends to be lower in total fat and saturated fat than dark meat.

Add variety by stocking up on fish and shellfish as a lower-fat alternative to other meats. Quality fish has a firm texture that springs back when pressed with your finger. Avoid anything with a fishy smell. Read the Nutrition Facts food label on breaded and battered fish products.

Choose processed and luncheon meats with the lowest fat content. Low-fat hot dogs, bologna, and bacon (traditional high-fat choices) can even be found. This category of products, however, tends to be higher in sodium.

Eggs

Buy eggs with the intention of using only the whites because all the fat is in the yolks.

Try low-fat and fat-free egg substitutes found in the refrigerated- and frozen-food sections.

Dairy

Milk comes in many forms—skim, low fat, reduced fat, whole—but for the least fat, choose skim or low-fat milk.

Compare labels on sour creams, dips, cottage cheeses, and yogurts; they vary in fat content. Some fat-free yogurts are made with artificial sweeteners, lowering the calorie count, too.

Most regular cheeses have about 9 fat grams per ounce, but there are many reduced-fat and fat-free products available in supermarkets. If you don't like the taste of one brand, don't get discouraged. On your next shopping trip, choose another brand. Some of the fat-free products are so good, they even melt like full-fat cheese.

Bakery

Breads fit in the base of the Food Guide Pyramid, so load up in this area of the store, too. Choose bread for sandwiches, bagels, dinner rolls, and bread sticks. Many stores that have their own bakery now offer fresh-baked breads with tempting flavors such as tomato basil, Italian garlic, and rosemary dill.

Muffins, bars, cakes, and danishes made in-house at the grocery store aren't required to be labeled with nutrition information, so buy with caution. Many regular muffins can have up to 20 fat grams each. You can, however, typically find reduced- or low-fat muffins and danishes in the bakery to satisfy your occasional craving for something sweet.

Angel food cake is always a fat-free choice, but be forewarned, it's loaded with calories just like all the other dessert choices.

Buying Frozen

Fruits and Vegetables

Most people believe that fresh is best when it comes to buying fruits and vegetables, but frozen is also a great choice. As soon as these products are harvested, they're flash frozen, holding in their flavor and nutrition. Whereas fresh may last only a few days before becoming overripe or rotting, frozen can last for months in your freezer. With frozen, you can take out only the amount you need for one meal or recipe and leave the rest in the freezer for another meal.

Read the Nutrition Facts on vegetables with sauces. Cheese and cream sauces can add fat.

Some fruits are frozen as is, but some have sugar added. The ingredient list will tell you if sugar has been added.

It's true that juices count toward your 5 servings a day, but it's typically better to eat the whole fruit or vegetable compared to the juice. Many juices, with the exception of citrus juices and others that have vitamins added, fall into the category of empty-calorie foods—choices that have calories, but not much else. When you do have juice, drink it in limited quantities and read food labels carefully to find those choices with the best nutritional value.

Frozen Meals

Look for dinners or entrées that have no more than 10 to 15 fat grams. For a balanced meal, add a bread, fruit or vegetable, and milk to these convenience products. Although many lower-fat dinner and meal options are available, they all tend to be high in sodium.

Desserts

Sorbets, sherbets, Italian ices, popsicles, low-fat or fat-free frozen yogurts, and ice cream are all good choices. As you shop, keep in mind the intended use of these products—as an occasional treat. Although these options may be low in fat, their calorie content is still high. Ice creams and yogurts have some calcium, but the level isn't high enough to position these desserts as a substitute for milk.

Buying Packaged

Bulk Bins

Foods in the bulk bins allow you to purchase just the amount you need, whether you're buying for one, two, or a house full of guests. The choices here tend to be less expensive than their brand name counterparts.

Canned Goods

Canned vegetables are higher in sodium than either fresh or frozen.

Some canned entrées, such as chili, spaghetti, or chow mein, can be low in fat. Always check the fat content on food labels.

Broth-based soups such as chicken noodle and vegetable beef are low fat. Cream soups tend to be higher in fat, but reduced-fat versions can be found on supermarket shelves. All soups are high in sodium.

Canned dried beans and legumes such as navy, pinto, and white northern beans offer much more convenience than the dried product. Loaded with fiber, these products work great in chili, homemade soups, and salads.

Dressings and Condiments

Naturally low-fat condiments include ketchup, salsa, mustard, Worcestershire sauce, barbecue sauce, and flavored vinegars.

Mayonnaise comes in reduced fat, low fat, and fat free. Find the balance of fat grams and taste that's right for you.

Salad dressings in every flavor—French, Italian, Thousand Island, ranch—come in fat-free varieties and actually taste as good as the full-fat version. Purchase these as a topping for pasta salads and baked potatoes in addition to vegetable salads.

Rice and Pasta

For variety, go beyond plain old pasta. Try different shapes and sizes, such as fusilli, cannelloni, or mini-lasagna noodles.

Brown rice has more fiber than white rice.

With the increasing popularity of ethnic foods, many different grains are available at supermarkets. Try couscous, barley, bulgur, or wild rice.

Convenience Products

Boxed rice, pasta, and potato dishes are available with a multitude of flavorings and sauces. Read the Nutrition Facts food label to find those lowest in fat and sodium. To cut the fat, consider skipping the margarine or butter called for in the recipe instructions when preparing these foods at home.

Cereals

Don't limit your purchases in this aisle to breakfast only. Cereal makes a great snack or a quick dinner. Most choices are naturally low fat—even low-fat granola cereals can be found.

Many cereals tend to be high in sugar. Choices lower in sugar contain 4 grams or less per serving. However, buying a low-sugar cereal isn't always the best choice if you add sugar at home in the bowl.

Cereal bars and toaster pastries are quick breakfast options when you have limited time, and most are fortified to have similar vitamins and minerals to cereals. Read the label for the fat grams and calories.

Snack Foods

Low-fat cracker choices include saltines, pretzels, graham crackers, and oyster crackers.

Fortune cookies, fig bars, and gingersnaps are lower-fat cookie choices.

Look for baked, oil-free potato and tortilla chips.

Although many low-fat and fat-free snack foods are available at the store, these products are not necessarily low in calories. Many of the reduced-fat products have almost as many calories as the traditional product.

A small handful of nuts or seeds has more than 20 fat grams. Reevaluate them as a snack food before purchasing.

Pantry Checklist

Before your next shopping trip, spend a few minutes taking stock of what's currently in your pantry. Jot down your favorite brands and products that fit into your meal plan for weight and diabetes management.

_____

_____

_____

_____

_____

My Stock up for Health Shopping List

_____

_____

_____

_____

_____

_____

_____

_____

_____

_____

_____

_____

_____

_____

_____

_____

Appendix C
The Low-Fat
Cooking Lesson

You don't have to be a registered dietitian or attend a gourmet cooking school to prepare delicious and nutritious meals. Cooking the enlightened way just takes practice. Use the Take Action Today tips provided here to lower the fat and retain the flavor in your favorite recipes. Experiment with the different suggestions to find a balance of flavor and health that suits your lifestyle. And remember, your taste buds will adjust, but you may have to try a new recipe ingredient a time or two before you begin favoring the new taste sensations.

Take Action Today

Try meatless entrées more often. Focus on pastas, grains, and vegetables instead of meat as the main component of meals.

Use less meat in casseroles, spaghetti, and chili. Add back texture with beans, mushrooms, onions, peppers, and grated carrots.

Experiment with fat-free yogurt, mashed bananas, or prune puree in place of some or all of the fat in quick bread and muffin recipes. There are several brands of commercial fruit purees available in grocery stores—they're convenient and serve the same purpose. Start by replacing half the fat with one of these substitutions and gradually increase the replacement amount as your tastes adjust. Be forewarned that the texture of these lighter products will be different than the traditional product (muffins may be more dense and not stay fresh for as many days, for example).

Leave out the margarine or butter and use skim milk when making convenience meals or side dishes such as macaroni and cheese, stuffing, or instant potatoes.

Try fat-free sandwich toppings such as mustard, ketchup, salsa, chutney, and barbecue sauce.

Choose light or reduced-fat margarines as a spread, but don't use them in your cookie recipes. These modified margarines have water whipped into them, which prevents cookies from turning out as they should (flatter, broader cookies, for example).

Consider how often you eat a food or make a recipe before you decide to modify it. If it's a meal you eat weekly, then making some fat-lowering changes is essential for healthful eating habits. Enjoy the original recipe of your favorite cake if you make it only on special occasions.

Experiment with fresh herbs and spices to add flavor to lean meats, salads, and sandwiches.

Use nonstick or Teflon pans instead of frying or sautéing in oil.

Beat egg whites slightly and use as a substitute for whole eggs in recipes.

On a regular basis, choose low-fat cooking methods such as steaming, grilling, microwaving, boiling, baking, or braising.

Cook, drain the grease, and rinse hamburger with hot water before adding it to sauce or seasoning it for tacos, spaghetti, or similar dishes.

Try flavored vinegars as a marinade for meats or as a salad dressing.

Make a substitute for sour cream or cream cheese by placing fat-free yogurt in a strainer lined with a coffee filter. Place a bowl under the strainer and refrigerate it for several hours or overnight. Liquid will drain out, leaving a thick yogurt cheese.

Use ground chicken or turkey in place of ground beef. Ground white meat poultry is the lowest in fat.

Homemade Turned Healthy

Cooking healthier doesn't mean you have to come up with totally new meals. Simple changes in your favorite recipes can be all it takes to stay within your fat gram budget. Remember, though, that some reduced-fat and fat-free ingredients may change your end product slightly. Fat-free cheese, for example, might not melt quite like full-fat cheese, and lightened-up baked goods may have a slightly different texture and may not stay fresh for as many days. But don't let that discourage you from making some changes—just make them gradually. Try the following suggestions the next time you're craving a home-cooked meal.

INSTEAD OF	TRY	FAT SAVINGS (gm)
margarine or butter	reduced-fat margarine	6 per tbsp.
whole milk	skim milk	8 per cup
oil	nonstick spray	25 per serving
mayonnaise	low-fat or fat-free mayonnaise	7–11 per tbsp.
sour cream	reduced-fat or fat-free sour cream	1–3 per tbsp.
cream cheese	reduced-fat, low-fat, fat-free cream cheese	4–9 per ounce
cheese	reduced-fat, low-fat, or fat-free cheese	4–9 per ounce
evaporated milk	evaporated skim milk	18 per cup
whole egg	egg substitute or 2 egg whites	5 per egg
ground beef	extra lean ground beef, ground turkey or chicken	11 per 3 oz.
poultry with the skin	skinless poultry	3–7 per piece
salad dressing	reduced-fat salad dressing	7 per tbsp.
mayonnaise, sour cream, cheese sauce, guacamole	ketchup, salsa, barbecue sauce, mustard	3–11 per tbsp.
double-crust pie	single-crust pie shell	60 per pie or 7 1/2 per 1/8th pie
shortening or oil	pureed prunes, prune baby food, mashed bananas, fat-free yogurt	200 per cup
margarine or butter	jams, jellies, apple butter	4 per tsp.
peanut butter	reduced-fat peanut butter	2–3 per tbsp.
cream soups	reduced-fat cream soups	5–10 per cup

How Simple It Is!

The following examples give you ideas on how to use the foregoing substitutions. Although several modifications are suggested for each sample recipe, you may want to try one or two changes first to see if your taste buds are satisfied. Once your likes have adjusted, consider making even further fat-lowering modifications. Remember, small, gradual changes are the key to long-term success.

Sample 1—Lasagna

TRADITIONAL	MODIFICATIONS
1 lb. ground beef	1 lb. ground turkey or chicken or extra lean ground beef (rinsed)
1/2 cup onion, chopped	
1 clove garlic, finely chopped	
1/2 tsp. salt	
1 can whole tomatoes, drained	
12 uncooked lasagna noodles	
16 oz. ricotta cheese	16 oz. fat-free ricotta cheese
1/2 cup grated Parmesan cheese	1/4 cup Parmesan cheese
2 cups shredded mozzarella cheese	1 1/2 cup low-fat mozzarella cheese
	add mushrooms and green peppers

Modifications made: used a lower-fat ground-beef replacement and lower-fat cheese, decreased amount of cheese in recipe, and added texture with additional vegetables. Fat savings: 120 grams per 9" × 13" pan of lasagna (or 15 grams per 1/8th pan).

Sample 2—Blueberry Muffins

TRADITIONAL	MODIFICATIONS
3/4 cup milk	3/4 cup skim milk
1/2 cup vegetable oil	1/2 cup prune baby food or fat-free yogurt
1 egg	2 egg whites, slightly beaten
2 cups flour	
1/3 cup sugar	
2 tsp. baking powder	
1/2 tsp. salt	
1 cup fresh or frozen blueberries	

Modifications made: used a nonfat milk, replaced vegetable oil, and tried egg whites in place of whole egg. Fat savings: 10 grams per muffin.

Sample 3—Cheesecake

TRADITIONAL	MODIFICATIONS
1 cup flour	
1/2 cup butter	6 tbsp. margarine
1/3 cup sugar	
1 egg yolk	
5 packages cream cheese	3 packages light cream cheese and 2 cups yogurt cheese
1 3/4 cup sugar	
3 tbsp. flour	
1 tbsp. grated lemon peel	
1/4 tsp. salt	
5 eggs	10 egg whites or equivalent egg substitute
2 egg yolks	
1/4 cup whipping cream	1/4 cup evaporated skim milk, whipped

Modifications made: eliminated egg yolks, used a lower-fat cream cheese and replaced some cream cheese, used nonfat evaporated milk. Fat savings: 230 grams per cheesecake (or 23 per 1/10th cake).

Resources

Chapter 1

"Novel Drugs for Type II Diabetes." *Harvard Health Letter* 21, no. 6 (April 1996): 4–6.

"Preventing Diabetes: The Wellness Plan." *UC Berkeley Wellness Letter,* November 1996.

"Standards of Medical Care for Patients With Diabetes Mellitus." *Diabetes Care* 20, suppl. (January 1997): S5–S13.

Wing, Rena R., et al. "Caloric Restriction Per Se Is a Significant Factor in Improvements in Glycemic Control and Insulin Sensitivity During Weight Loss in Obese NIDDM Patients." *Diabetes Care* 17, no. 1 (January 1994): 30–36.

Chapter 2

Agras, W. Stewart. "Treatment of the Obese Binge Eater." In *Eating Disorders and Obesity,* edited by Brownell, Kelly D. and Christopher G. Fairburn. New York: Guilford Press, 1995.

Chisholm, D. N., et al. "Physical Activity Readiness." *British Columbia Medical Journal* 17 (1975): 375–78.

Fairburn, Christopher G., and G. Terence Wilson. "Binge Eating: Definition and Classification." In *Binge Eating: Nature, Assessment, and*

Treatment, edited by Fairburn, Christopher G. and G. Terence Wilson. New York: Guilford Press, 1993.

Meisler, Jodi Godfrey, and Sachiko St. Jeor. "Summary and Recommendations From the American Health Foundation's Expert Panel on Healthy Weight." *American Journal of Clinical Nutrition* 63, suppl. (1996): 474S–77S.

"The New Diet Pills: Fairly (But Not Completely) Safe." *Harvard Heart Letter* 7, no. 4 (December 1996): 1–2.

"Position of The American Dietetic Association: Weight Management." *Journal of The American Dietetic Association* 97, no. 1 (January 1997): 71–74.

U.S. Department of Agriculture, Agricultural Research Service, Dietary Guidelines Advisory Committee. *Report of the Dietary Guidelines Advisory Committee on the Dietary Guidelines for Americans, 1995*. Washington, D.C., 1995.

Weight Loss Readiness Quiz. Nutrition Fact Sheet: National Center for Nutrition and Dietetics.

Chapter 3

American Dietetic Association. *Nutrition Practice Guidelines for Type I and Type II Diabetes Mellitus*. The American Dietetic Association, 1996.

Carlson, Sydne K. "The Effect of Different Foods on Postprandial Blood Glucose Excursions." *On the Cutting Edge* 17, no. 4 (summer 1996): 11–12.

Franz , Marion J. "Nutrition Principles for the Management of Diabetes and Related Complications." *Diabetes Care* 17, no. 5 (May 1994) 490–518.

"Nutrition Recommendations and Principles for People With Diabetes Mellitus." *Diabetes Care* 20, suppl. (January 1997): S14–S17.

"Nutrition Recommendations and Principles for People With Diabetes Mellitus." *Journal of The American Dietetic Association* 94, no. 5 (May 1994): 504–11.

Pascal, Randy W., et al. "Effects of a Behavioral Weight Loss Program Stressing Calorie Restriction Versus Calorie Plus Fat Restriction in Obese Individuals With NIDDM or a Family History of Diabetes." *Diabetes Care* 18, no. 9 (September 1995): 1241–48.

"Position of The American Dietetic Association: Use of Nutritive and Nonnutritive Sweeteners." *Journal of The American Dietetic Association* 93, no. 7 (July 1993): 816–21.

United States Department of Agriculture. *The Food Guide Pyramid.* 1992.

Chapter 4

"Exercise." In *A Core Curriculum for Diabetes Education.* 2d ed. Chicago: American Association of Diabetes Educators, 1993.

"Foot Care in Patients With Diabetes Mellitus." *Diabetes Care* 19, suppl. (January 1996): S23–S24.

U.S. Department of Health and Human Services. *Physical Activity and Health: A Report of the Surgeon General.* Atlanta: U.S. Department of Health and Human Services, Centers for Disease Control and Prevention, National Center for Chronic Disease Prevention and Health Promotion, 1996.

Chapter 5

"Monitoring and Management." In *A Core Curriculum for Diabetes Education.* 2d ed. Chicago: American Association of Diabetes Educators, 1993.

"Standards of Medical Care for Patients With Diabetes Mellitus." *Diabetes Care* 20, suppl. 1 (January 1997): S5–S13.

"Tests of Glycemia in Diabetes." *Diabetes Care* 20, suppl. 1 (January 1997): S18–S21,.

Wylie-Rosett, Judith, et al. "Comprehensive Monitoring for Evaluating Diabetes Therapy." In *Handbook of Diabetes Medical Nutrition Therapy.* Gaithersburg, MD, Aspen Publishers, 1996.

Chapter 6

Mackenzie, Alec. *Time for Success: A Goal Getter's Strategy.* New York: McGraw-Hill Publishing Co., 1989.

Chapter 7

Greene, Geoffrey W., et al. "Stages of Change for Reducing Dietary Fat to 30% of Energy or Less." *Journal of The American Dietetic Association* 94, no. 9 (October 1994): 1105–10.

Invest in Your Health Weight Control. Minneapolis: University of Minnesota, 1987.

Prochaska, James O. *Changing for Good.* New York: William Morrow, 1994.

Sandoral, Wendy M. "Stages of Change: A Model for Nutrition Counseling." *Topics in Clinical Nutrition* 9, no. 3 (1994): 64–69.

Chapter 8

Olesen, Erik. *Twelve Steps to Mastering the Winds of Change: Peak Performers Reveal How to Stay on Top in Times of Turmoil.* New York: Macmillan, 1993.

Parham, Ellen S. "Enhancing Social Support in Weight Loss Management Groups." *Journal of The American Dietetic Association* 93, no. 10 (October 1993): 1152–56.

Chapter 9

"Diabetes Mellitus and Exercise." *Diabetes Care* 20, suppl. (January 1997): S51.

"Exercise." In *A Core Curriculum for Diabetes Education.* 2d ed. Chicago: American Association of Diabetes Educators, 1993.

Franz, Marion J. "Exercise Benefits and Guidelines for Persons With Diabetes." In *Handbook of Diabetes Medical Nutrition Therapy,* Gaithersburg, MD.: Aspen Publishers, 1996.

Hayes, Charlotte. "Pattern Management: A Tool for Improving Blood Glucose Control With Exercise." *On the Cutting Edge* 17, no. 4 (summer 1996): 4–7.

Invest in Your Health Weight Control. Minneapolis: University of Minnesota, 1987.

Sexton, Amy. "Weight Training: A Great Way to Burn Calories." *Personal Weight Management* 1, no. 2 (August 1996): 5.

U.S. Department of Health and Human Services. *Physical Activity and Health: A Report of the Surgeon General.* Atlanta: U.S. Department of Health and Human Services, Centers for Disease Control and Prevention, National Center for Chronic Disease Prevention and Health Promotion, 1996.

Zelasko, Chester J. "Exercise for Weight Loss: What Are the Facts?" *Journal of The American Dietetic Association* 95, no. 12 (December 1995): 1414–17.

Chapter 10

Alcohol, Alcohol Everywhere, but Is It Safe to Drink? American Diabetes Association, 1995.

Facts About Fat Substitutes. National Center for Nutrition and Dietetics, 1994.

Franz, Marion J., et al. "Nutrition Principles for the Management of Diabetes and Related Complications." *Diabetes Care* 17, no. 5 (May 1994): 490–518.

Gershoff, Stanley N. "Nutrition Evaluation of Dietary Fat Substitutes." *Nutrition Reviews* 53, no. 11 (November 1995): 305–13.

Guidelines for Use of Alcohol in Diabetes. Twin Cities District Dietetic Association Diet Manual, 1994.

"Nutrition Recommendations and Principles for People With Diabetes Mellitus." *Diabetes Care* 17, no. 5 (May 1994): 519–22.

Schmidt, Lois E. "Practical Mineral Recommendations: Translation to Clinical Practice," *The Diabetes Educator* 21, no. 1 (January/February 1995): 21–23.

Chapter 11

Brown, Mona Boyd. *Label Facts for Healthful Eating—Educator's Resource Guide.* Dayton: The Mazer Corporation, 1993.

Chapter 12

Food Guide Pyramid With Popular Chinese Fare. The American Dietetic Association, 1995.

Food Guide Pyramid With Popular Italian Fare. The American Dietetic Association, 1995.

Food Guide Pyramid With Popular Mexican Fare. The American Dietetic Association, 1995.

Kulkarni, Karmeen D. "Adjusting Nutrition Therapy for Special Situations." *In Handbook of Diabetes Medical Nutrition Therapy.* Gaithersburg, Md.: Aspen Publishers, 1996.

Nutrition Practice Guidelines for Type I and Type II Diabetes Mellitus. The American Dietetic Association, 1996.

Roth, Harriet. *Guide to Low-Cholesterol Dining Out.* New York: Penguin, 1990.

Chapter 13

Brownell, Kelly D. *The LEARN Program for Weight Control.* University of Pennsylvania School of Medicine, 1988.

Brownell, Kelly D., et al. "Understanding and Preventing Relapse." *American Psychologist,* July 1986, 765–82.

"Mindfulness and Metaphor in Relapse Prevention: An Interview With G. Alan Marlatt." *Journal of The American Dietetic Association* 94, no. 8 (August 1994): 846–48.

Chapter 14

Braham, Barbara J. *Managing Stress: Keeping Calm Under Fire.* Burr Ridge, IL.: Irwin Professional Publishing, 1994.

Common Sense About Feeling Tense, American Heart Association Heart At Work Program Module. Dallas, 1995.

Davis, Martha, et al. *The Relaxation and Stress Reduction Workbook.* Oakland: New Harbinger Publications, 1995.

Gawain, Shakti. *Creative Visualization.* San Rafael, CA: New World Library, 1995.

Helmstetter, Shad. *The Self-Talk Solution*. New York: Pocket Books, 1987.

Ornish, Dean. *Dr. Dean Ornish's Program for Reversing Heart Disease*. Random House, 1990.

Warpeha, Annette, and Jeanette Harris. "Combining Traditional and Nontraditional Approaches to Nutrition Counseling." *Journal of The American Dietetic Association* 93, no. 7 (July 1993): 797–800.

"What Stress Does to Diabetes Control." *Diabetes Forecast*, December 1995.

Appendix A

Fast Food Facts. Minnesota Attorney General's Office.

Nutritionist IV, version 3.0, N2 Computing.

Appendix B

Grocery Buying Guide. American Heart Association, Minnesota Affiliate, 1994.

Supermarket Nutrition Shopping for Good Health. The American Dietetic Association, 1995.

Index

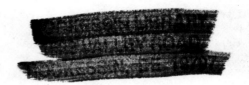
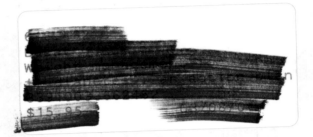